Diets in a Nutshell

A Definitive Guide on Diets from A to Z

Mary Josephine Scales

Apex Publishers

Clifton, Virginia

Diets in a Nutshell

A Definitive Guide on Diets from A to Z
By Mary Josephine Scales

Credits

Editor: Ted Goldammer
Cover Design: Torie Goldammer

Apex Publishers

email: customer-serivce@apexpublishers.com
http://www.apexpublishers.com

Notice of Rights

Notice of Liability

Publisher's Cataloging-In-Publication Data
(Prepared by The Donohue Group, Inc.)

Scales, Mary Josephine.
   Diets in a nutshell : definitive guide on diets from A to Z / Mary Josephine Scales.
   p. ; cm.
   Includes index.
   ISBN: 0-9675212-1-1
1. Dietetics. 2. Reducing diets--Evaluation. 3. Diet Fads--Evaluation. 4. Diet therapy--Evaluation. 5. Nutrition. 6. Consumer education. I. Title.
RM216 .S253 2005
613.2   2005929790

Printed and bound in the United States of America.

Dedication

To my husband Robert and to all my wonderful children and
grandchildren.

Michael
Robin
Teddy
Jeff
Benjamin
Ché
Gina
Jeff
Jill
Joseph
Kelsey
Kevin
Kyle
Lucas
Nathan
Patrick
Torie

Contents

Section II: Diets for Medical Conditions

Section III: Diets by Health & Government Organizations

Preface

Almost everyone at one time or another has gone on a diet. The motivation to diet can be for medical reasons or for the interests of vanity. Although some of these diets are based on good science and are safe and effective, some are useless, untested, or even dangerous. Desperate dieters, however, are easily seduced by anecdotal accounts of quick weight loss or promises of early success. With so much propaganda—not to mention the number of diets on the market today—it can be a difficult task for anyone to choose the best diet.

Diets in a Nutshell is intended as a definitive up-to-date guide that reviews many of the diet plans on the market today. The material in the book has been arranged into three broad sections: fad diets, diets for medical conditions, and diets by major health or government organizations. Within these sections, topics are well organized and indexed.

Although there are literally hundreds of fad diets, Section I reviews some of the more popular diets, such as the Atkins Diet, the Cabbage Soup Diet, and the Zone Diet. Typically fad diets make promises of improved health, greater life expectancy, and/or weight loss. While some of these diets are recommended by nutritionists, others can seriously undermine your health. In Section I, the more popular diets are reviewed in very general terms. For each diet an overview will be given, then an explanation of how it works and an examination of its strengths and weaknesses, followed by an overall assessment of the diet. The overview, how it works and its strengths are the opinion of the author, while its weaknesses and the overall assessment of the diet is based on the opinions of nutritionists. Section II focuses on diets for specific medical conditions, such as acid reflux, diabetes, attention deficit disorder, premenstrual symptoms, irritable bowel syndrome, or prostate cancer. Diets for specific medical conditions reflect the opinions of medical experts in their respective fields. Section III discusses those diets that have been recommended by major health and government organizations.

A word of warning: It's always best to seek the advice of a registered dietitian or a physician before undertaking any diet plan.

Introduction

There are many diets to choose from in today's society. Some require extreme reductions in the number of calories consumed, others rely on supplements alleged to help burn fat, and still others are based on eating a single type of food. Some of these diets advocate eating only those foods that your ancestors could have hunted or gathered, as with the Caveman Diet. While other diets claim that to lose weight you must eat foods in certain combinations or limit your choices according to your blood type or temporarily fast, as with the Detox Diet. A number of diets, such as the Atkins Diet, claim that carbohydrates cause weight gain, so they stress eating protein-rich foods with little regard to fat content. Still other diet plans present an opposite argument, urging you to eat a low-fat, high-carbohydrate diet. There are also various types of vegetarian diets, ranging from those that allow fish, eggs, or dairy, to those that allow no animal products at all. With so many conflicting viewpoints, it can be difficult to determine which diet is the best for you.

The motivation to diet can be for health reasons, but more typically one goes on a diet to lose weight because of social pressures. The view of society that "thin is in" has contributed to the obsession of weight loss. People are often willing to try anything that promises weight loss, and companies that promote fad diets take advantage of this fact. Many diets appeal to people by promising quick and easy weight loss, avoiding the effort to lose weight through long-term changes in their eating and exercise habits.

Promoting diets and diet products is a major industry in the United States with Americans spending an estimated $50 billion a year feeding the weight-loss industry. This figure includes money spent on diet centers and programs; prepackaged diet foods; over-the-counter and prescription diet drugs; weight-loss books and magazines; physicians, nurses, nutritionists, and other health professionals specializing in weight-loss; commercial and residential exercise clubs with weight-loss programs; and food products that are sugar-free, fat-free, and reduced calorie ("lite") food products and sugar substitutes.

While weight loss diets and products long have been promoted as a permanent cure for obesity, they rarely produce long-lasting results. According to medical research, only a small percentage of dieters succeed in losing a significant amount of weight and maintaining that loss over a long-term period. In fact a large percentage of all dieters regain some—if not all—of the weight originally lost, and in some cases gain even more weight. In recent years, an increasing body of research has substantiated this diet failure rate and acknowledges obesity can be caused by a combination of factors, including social, cultural, genetic, physiologic, metabolic, behavioral and psychological issues.

For years, the commercial weight loss industry was largely unregulated. Only recently, due to Congressional pressure, have the Federal Trade Commission (FTC) and the Food and Drug Administration (FDA) begun to enforce existing regulations. However, many of these regulations are narrow in scope and only loosely enforced. They could go much further in protecting the public health.

SECTION I

Fad Diets

The Abs Diet

Overview

The Abs Diet, popularized by the best-selling book *The Abs Diet: The Six-Week Plan to Flatten Your Stomach and Keep You Lean for Life* by David Zinczenko, is not just for athletes, models, body builders, or trainers, but for the average person also. The fundamental principle of the Abs Diet is to build up the muscles in the abdomen to speed up the losing of health-hazardous belly fat. Zinczenko says that for every pound of muscle gained, dieters need 50 extra calories per day just to maintain the added muscle.

Zinczenko says his diet is capable of widespread success because it isn't about losing weight and restricting foods, but about gaining a healthy life-style and body.

How it Works

The Abs Diet prescribes eating six evenly spaced meals and two snacks per day around the Abs Diet 12 Power Foods. Zinczenko says eating evenly spaced meals is better at maintaining your "energy balance." People with large energy imbalances (those with large calorie surpluses or shortfalls) are generally more overweight, while those with the most balanced energy levels are the leanest. The idea is to eat regularly so that you never go hungry and gorge.

The Abs Diet encourages you to focus on (not restrict yourself to) a generous market basket of food types—the Abs Diet 12 Power Foods—to fulfill your core nutritional needs. It focuses on using 12 Power Foods in the meal plans, which provide all the vitamins, minerals and fiber you need for good health, while promoting muscle growth and fat burning.

There is less emphasis on the number of calories consumed than with other diets since the 12 Power Foods will really help self-regulate your calorie consumption. So, if you get enough protein, fiber, and good carbohydrates, in essence your body will "count" your calories for you.

Zinczenko says the more of the 12 Power Foods you eat, the better your body will be able to increase lean muscle mass and avoid storing fat. He recommends including two or three of the 12 Power foods in each of your three major meals and at least one of them in each of your three smaller snacks. He also says it's important to diversify your food at every meal to get a combination of protein, carbohydrates and fat and to make sure you sneak a little bit of protein into each snack.

The 12 Power Foods consist of almonds and other nuts, beans and other legumes, spinach and other green vegetables, low-fat dairy products, instant hot oatmeal, eggs, turkey and other lean meats, peanut butter, olive oil, whole-grain breads and cereals, Extra-Protein (whey) Powder, and raspberries and other berries.

The Abs Diet recommends avoiding the following foods: salted foods, meats that are high in saturated fats (like sausage, bacon, cured meats and fatty cuts of steak (like T-bone and rib-eye), breakfast cereals that are high in sugar, whole milk and (in some cases) frozen yogurt, trans-fatty foods (margarine, fried foods, and commercially manufactured baked goods), hydrogenated vegetable oils, and processed bakery products like white bread, bagels and doughnuts. It also suggests restricting alcohol consumption to two to three drinks per week.

The Diet does allow cheating for one meal each week, which is designed to reward you for good work throughout the week, and help keep cravings in check. Zinczenko believes that the best way to control cravings is to satisfy them every so often.

The exercise component begins in week three of the six-week plan and includes a 20-minute full-body workout three days a week. It also includes regular strength training, brisk walking or other aerobic exercises and, of course, some detailed abdominal work—50 core exercises in five regions of the abdomen.

Advantages

- The Abs Diet builds muscle.
- The Diet helps promote weight loss.
- The Diet also strengthens bones, lowers blood pressure, fights cancer, and minimizes the risk of heart disease.

Disadvantages

- The prominence of packaged foods recommended by the Abs Diet does conflict with the book's advice on limiting sodium to keep blood pressure low.

Summary

Even though some diets can be unhealthy, the Abs Diet has some good positive messages for dieters to take with them. This diet and exercise plan—aimed mainly at men—promotes healthy fats, protein and calcium consumption, all of which are staples of a balanced diet. However, nutritional experts raise questions about the use of protein powder. Although preliminary studies suggest dieters might benefit from a diet that's a little higher in protein than usual, people can get extra protein just as easily by having some light cottage cheese or a few additional ounces of lean meat or fish.

Anne Collins Diet

Overview

The Anne Collins Diet, created by nutritionist and weight loss consultant Anne Collins, is a low-priced online weight loss program that includes a variety of flexible diet plans to suit most dieters. All the diet plans include ordinary foods that can be purchased in any grocery store. The diet plans are simple to follow, with a lot of useful information.

How it Works

All Collins' diet plans are based on healthy eating and can be adjusted to almost any calorie intake between 1,100 and 3,000 calories per day. They include a complete set of menus with the focus on easy-to-cook convenience meals, with a range of fast-food options. The calorie content of all foods is displayed, so dieters see exactly what they are eating and learn what foods to eat in the future.

The Anne Collins program also offers a 365-day email support helpline.

In general the diet plans are not complicated and should be easy to follow. To date Anne Collins offers nine diet plans, which are:

1. Low Carb Diet
2. Balanced Weight Loss Diet
3. Low Calorie Weight Loss Diet
4. Low Glycemic Weight Loss Diet
5. Cholesterol-Lowering Weight Loss Diet
6. Vegetarian Quick-Start Diet
7. 10-Minute Meals Diet
8. Diet for Life
9. Vegetarian Diet for Life

The Low Carb Diet is a reduced-carbohydrate eating plan that allows you to lose up to 10 pounds in the first two weeks, and to continue losing weight in a fast healthy way until you reach your goal. The plan is designed to help you reduce cravings and lose weight as fast as possible. It is packed with quick and easy low-carbohydrate meals using ordinary foods.

The Balanced Weight Loss Diet is a 28-day weight loss plan with a wide range of quick, nutritious meals, a choice of calorie-controlled snacks including candy, cookies, and wine and beer to choose from. Fast food, frozen entrees, and "take-to-work" lunches are all part of this easy to follow diet. It's extremely flexible—you can even add extra snacks to increase your calories according to how quickly you want to lose weight.

The Low Calorie Booster Diet is a complete eating plan with two alternative 14-day menu plans for maximum choice. Each day, the diet offers three meals and three snacks to make sure you eat small amounts of food and often in order to speed up your metabolism. It is designed only for short-term use to increase weight loss.

The Low Glycemic Diet is designed for dieters, like diabetics, who wish to lose weight and reduce their intake of refined or high-glycemic carbohydrates. This diet is designed to help you reduce cravings and lose weight at the fastest possible speed. The Low Glycemic Diet also helps dieters who suffer from hypothyroidism or fluctuating blood sugar levels.

The Cholesterol-Lowering Diet is a low-fat eating plan that allows you to lose 10 pounds a month, and to go on losing weight in a fast healthy way until you reach your goal. The diet is designed to help you reduce cholesterol, improve your heart health and normalize your weight at the fastest possible speed. It is packed with delicious meals, using ordinary foods.

The Vegetarian Quick-Start Diet is designed mainly for ovo-lacto vegetarians but it's adaptable for all vegetarians, including vegans. Weight loss will average about 10 pounds a month or more if you have a lot of weight to lose.

The 10-Minute Meals Diet is a 28-day eating plan that (as the name suggests) provides a wide choice of healthy meals that may be cooked in 10 minutes or less. The plan includes meals that can be prepared and cooked quickly, microwave meals, fast-food options, and meals that may be cooked and eaten over two days. To make dieting even easier, this plan provides a wide range of quick-to-prepare take-to-work meals.

The Diet for Life Diet is a healthy, balanced, low-fat eating plan that includes over 80 easy main meal recipes for all the family to enjoy. The Vegetarian Diet for Life Diet is a healthy vegetarian plan that includes over 120 main meal recipes for all the family to enjoy. These plans include meals for one, two, or four people and a great range of recipes for soups, desserts, and smoothies. They also include advice on how to read labels, shopping and dining out. These diets are an ideal way to maintain good health and a great shape for life.

Advantages

- The Anne Collins Diet is easy to follow and relatively inexpensive.
- The meals are wide ranging and taste good, and ingredients can be purchased at any grocery store.
- The plan teaches how to modify your eating habits on a long-term basis.
- Great advice on diet motivation is offered by the online support network.
- Extra motivation is also available, which can help people who begin to fall by the wayside.

Disadvantages

- The Anne Collins Diet doesn't emphasize exercise enough.

Summary

The Anne Collins Diet is one of the better weight loss plans on the market. It focuses on eating healthy and changing your attitude about food. But it downplays the importance of exercise in an all-out effort to get you to focus on eating better. For sustained weight loss, the best diet is usually a balanced diet with foods from all the nutritional food groups, which offers realistic weight reduction goals and provides a manageable eating plan. For most people, purely focusing on food is the problem in the first place, regardless of whether the food was healthy or unhealthy. Exercise is the one thing in common with all those who lose weight and keep it off.

3

Atkins Diet

Overview

The most widely used high-protein diet is the one advocated by the late Robert C. Atkins, M.D., of New York City. His 1972 book *Dr. Atkins' Diet Revolution* sold millions of copies in the first two years. His 1992 update, *Dr. Atkins' New Diet Revolution*, has sold even more. His low-carbohydrate, high-fat/high-protein weight loss approach focuses on the consumption of nutrient-dense, unprocessed foods (foods high in protein and fat) and vitamin-nutrient supplementation. The Atkins Diet specifically recommends animal proteins, therefore this isn't a diet for vegetarians. There is no hunger between meals since there are no limits on the amount of calories or quantities of foods allowed on the diet (e.g., meat, cheese, and eggs).

The Atkins theory is that excess carbohydrate intake (such as potatoes, fruit, bread, rice, pasta and other cereal foods) prevents the body from burning fat efficiently. Atkins claims that drastically reducing the daily intake of carbohydrates will remove toxins from your body, stabilize blood sugar, and rid yourself of fatigue, irritability, depression, headaches, and joint pain.

Atkins believes that if you severely restrict carbohydrate intake, your body will be forced to use extra fat deposits for energy. During the process of converting fat to energy, the body produces an abundance of substances called ketones, which are believed to suppress appetite. This "ketosis," as it is called, is central to the Atkins weight-loss plan.

How it Works

There are four phases to the Atkins Diet: (1) The Induction Phase, which switches your body to fat-burning from carbohydrate burning; (2) the Ongoing Weight Loss Phase or actual weight loss phase; (3) the Pre-Maintenance Phase, which is the transition phase from weight loss to maintaining your new optimum weight; and (4) the Lifetime Maintenance Phase, which maintains your healthy weight. Atkins Diet food selections differ to varying degrees depending upon the phase you are in and your individual metabolism. Atkins also recommended large amounts of nutritional supplements.

Atkins recommends that you regularly test your urine for ketones, which you can do yourself using a litmus-type paper that's available from most drug stores. If your urine tests negative for ketones, then you haven't cut back on your carbohydrates enough.

Induction Phase (Phase I)

The first phase of the Atkins Diet is the induction phase, which is designed to rebalance an individual's metabolism. The induction phase is designed to switch your body from burning carbohydrate to primarily burning fat for energy which will help you to lose weight and control your appetite. It lasts for 14 days and has strict restrictions on particular foods for the body to trigger ketosis. During this phase of the Atkins Diet, unlimited amounts of fat and protein are allowed, but the consumption of carbohydrates is restricted to only 15 to 20 grams per day. Foods allowed include butter, oil, meat, poultry, fish, eggs, cheese, and cream. Carbohydrates are obtained primarily from salads and other non-starchy vegetables, not from bread, rise, potatoes, sugar, or even fruit.

Ongoing Weight Loss Phase (Phase II)

Once you have completed the induction phase of Atkins Diet, you are ready for the second phase: the ongoing weight loss phase. During this phase weight loss is slower, and some foods are allowed back into the diet. Carbohydrates are added back into the diet, in the form of nutrient-dense and fiber-rich foods, by increasing to 25 grams daily the first week, 30 grams daily the next week, and so on until weight loss stops. Then you subtract carbohydrates from your daily intake in 5-gram increments so that you continue sustained, moderate weight loss.

In this phase, you can probably move beyond vegetables to food like nuts, berries, and possibly whole grain. When you are about 10 pounds from the desired weight, you can begin the pre-maintenance phase.

Pre-Maintenance Phase (Phase III)

When you reach the pre-maintenance phase it means you are between five and 10 pounds away from your target weight. The weight loss now is very slow. More foods are re-introduced into your diet. You increase your carbohydrate intake by 10-gram increments each week as long as you continue to lose weight. When you reach your goal weight, you stay at that level for a month before increasing your carbohydrate consumption. You can then increase your carbohydrate consumption by another 10 grams each week to see if you can consume that level without gaining weight. If you begin to gain weight, you cut back the weekly intake of carbohydrates by 10 grams, and you have established your Critical Carbohydrate Level for Maintenance and are ready for lifetime maintenance.

Lifetime Maintenance Phase (Phase IV)

The final phase of the Atkins Diet, the lifetime maintenance phase, is designed to maintain your target weight. Dieters following this low carbohydrate diet are encouraged to stick with the fourth phase diet for life in order to remain healthy and avoid gaining weight. At this stage, carbohydrate intake will be around 40 to 60 grams daily, depending on the individual.

Nutrient Supplementation

Adherence to the Atkins Diet can result in vitamin and mineral deficiencies. Atkins recommends a wide-range of nutritional supplements, including a multi-vitamin to correct any nutritional deficiencies that may occur while on the diet. Among his recommendations, Atkins suggests the following daily dosages: 300–600 micrograms (mcg) of chromium picolinate, 100–

400 milligrams (mg) of pantetheine, 200 mcg of selenium, and 450–675 mcg of biotin. At the very least, you'll need a daily multi-vitamin and about 1,000 milligrams of calcium to make up for what the diet lacks.

Advantages

- The Atkins Diet is believed to lower risk for chronic illnesses, like heart disease, high blood pressure, and diabetes.

- The primary benefit of the diet is rapid and substantial weight loss. Initially, much of the weight loss is due to water loss. Long-term weight loss occurs because with a low amount of carbohydrate intake, the body burns stored fat for energy.

- Because you can eat as much as you like of the permitted foods, you don't get hungry.

- It is argued that a low carbohydrate diet is more natural for the human body because grains in the form of wheat and rice were not part of our diet until about 10,000 years ago. Atkins claims our bodies have not evolved enough to cope with grains satisfactorily.

- Some research indicates that people with Type Two diabetes have better insulin function and better blood sugar control on a low carbohydrate diet.

- The diet is considered good for managing many health disorders, including headaches, blood sugar disorders, food intolerances, allergies, and many other health problems.

Disadvantages

- The Atkins Diet doesn't conform to the American Heart Association's dietary guidelines for a healthy heart.

- Any diet that limits carbohydrates causes the body to rely on fat or muscle for energy. When our body breaks down stored fat to supply energy, byproducts called ketones are formed. Ketones suppress appetite, but they also cause fatigue, nausea, and potentially dangerous fluid loss. In sever cases it can cause unconsciousness and even lead to a coma. Anyone with diabetes, or heart or kidney problems should NOT follow a diet that promotes the formation of ketones.

- People with diabetes taking insulin are at risk of becoming hypoglycemic if they do not eat appropriate carbohydrates.

- People who exercise regularly may experience low energy levels and muscle fatigue from low carbohydrate intake.

- The Atkins Diet is not recommended for pregnant women or nursing mothers, or for people being treated for high blood pressure.

- Eating unlimited amounts of fat, especially saturated fat found in meat products, can lead to increased risk of heart disease in the long term.

- High-protein diets also flush calcium out in the urine, which is bad for bones.

- Restricting carbohydrates means eating a low-fiber diet, which can cause constipation.

- Extensive research on healthy populations tells us to eat more fruits, vegetables, and whole grains. Diets low in carbohydrates may be lacking in some vitamins, minerals, and antioxidants.

- Studies show that restrictive diets, which eliminate several foods or food groups, have the worst failure rates over time—a pretty dismal outlook.

- One unattractive feature is that the diet can also cause bad breath. This is a result of ketosis—the state the body goes into during starvation.

Summary

Nutritionists generally balk at the idea of high-protein diets and argue that the Atkins Diet has not been proven effective for long-term weight loss. They are critical of the diet's focus on high protein, which emphasizes foods like meat and eggs that are high in cholesterol and saturated fats and low in fiber. Most nutritionists agree that Americans already eat more protein and fat than their bodies need, and eating a high-protein, high-fat diet raises the risk of many types of disease. The most serious claim against the Atkins Diet is that it's linked to a number of potential health risks such as osteoporosis, stroke, coronary heart disease, a propensity to form kidney stones, liver disorders, and diabetes.

They are also critical that the diet discourages eating many of the foods and food groups called for in the USDA Food Guide, such as fruits, cereals, grains, and vegetables.

4

Beverly Hills Diet

Overview

The Beverly Hills Diet, the brainchild of Judy Mazel, is a food combining weight loss plan that relies heavily on fruits. Mazel advocates a practice she terms "Cautious Combining." "It is when you eat and what foods you eat together that matters," she claims. According to Mazel, the enzymes necessary for digestion are found in the foods themselves, and each form of food contains the enzymes that allow that food to be digested in the intestine. Thus, each of the three food groups—proteins, carbohydrates and fats—contains their own set of enzymes to break down food so that the body can properly digest it. Mazel believes the enzymes in each specific fruit, along with the combination of foods eaten are critical to the success of her diet. Furthermore, enzymes from one food can't "cross over" to work on other food groups. Mazel also believes that when enzymes cross over it leads to enzyme confusion, and consequently the foods are not properly digested, and the undigested food is converted to fat and stored in the body.

How it Works

The diet begins with a 35-day plan that specifies items to be eaten at each meal, without counting calories or fat grams. In the first 10 days, only fruit is permitted. On day 11, carbohydrates and butter are added, and on day 19, protein is added. Fatty treats are permitted. Mazel recommends eating fruit by itself and never eating protein with carbohydrates, so the food can be properly digested and not stored as fat. Mazel says you'll lose 10 to 15 pounds in 35 days by following rules on eating specific foods at the same time or in a certain order each day.

Advantages

- The Beverly Hills Diet can prevent disease.
- Initial weight loss can be rapid.

- Many people like following a very structured menu plan.

Disadvantages

- The Beverly Hills Diet relies on extremely limiting meal guidelines and is not based on any scientific evidence.
- Critics of the diet say that eating so little protein can lead to protein deficiency and consequently a loss in lean muscle rather than fat.
- Too much fruit; not only is this diet plan monotonous, but also it results in an inadequate intake of protein and fat, as well as iron, zinc, vitamin B12, calcium, and essential fatty acids. It is almost universally agreed that humans need a wide variety of foods to obtain the huge range of essential nutrients and other health-promoting constituents of food (such as antioxidants) that promote optimal health.
- Weight loss is hard to maintain.
- The diet doesn't teach you how to eat properly.
- The diet fails to tackle the issue of portion control or exercise, both of which are directly relevant to any successful weight loss program.
- Mazel encourages consuming a single food, grapes for example, for an entire day, which is not only nutritionally inadequate but also boring.

Summary

The Beverley Hills Diet is a very unbalanced way of eating and cannot be recommended for even short periods (e.g., during weight loss), let alone as a lifelong diet. Food-combining diet plans are not established as an effective weight loss method. In spite of Mazel's claims, medical experts argue that all foods (except plain sugar) are a mixture of carbohydrates, protein, and fat and the body produces all the enzymes needed to digest foods without complicated food-combining plans. Also, medical experts have been quick to point out that Mazel's claim that undigested food is converted to fat is inaccurate. Doctors say undigested food that is not absorbed cannot be metabolized, and thereby passes through the digestive tract to the large intestine where it is broken down by bacteria, forms gas, or is eliminated as body waste.

Mazel, like Atkins, neglects to address portion control and serving sizes, concepts central to any serious program of long-term weight management. Perhaps most puzzling, however, is Mazel's silence on the subject of exercise. Regular physical activity is crucial for losing and maintaining weight, but the closest Mazel gets to this topic is her admonition to chew food thoroughly. The best way to lose excess fat and maintain a healthy weight in the long term is to follow a balanced calorie-controlled diet and do regular aerobic exercise and or weight resistance training.

5

Blood Type Diet

Overview

The Blood Type Diet, popularized by the best-selling book *Eat Right For Your Type* by Dr. Peter D'Adamo, a naturopathic physician, is based on the theory that people with different blood types respond differently to specific foods. According to D'Adamo, your blood type is the key to weight gain, as well as to health, disease, longevity, vitality, emotional strength, and personality. D'Adamo's ideas are rooted in evolutionary history, and, specifically, the observation that different blood types (Type O, Type A, Type B, and Type AB) came into existence at different stages during human cultural development. As a result, he believes that the key to optimal health is to eat as our ancestors with the same blood type did. Eating foods that are incompatible with your blood type poses considerable health risks, according to D'Adamo's theory. Type O's for instance, are descended from hunters and consequently must eat meat to maintain optimum health and to lose weight. Type A's, on the other hand, are vegetarians.

Whether a blood type is compatible with a food or not depends on a factor called lectins, which are low carbohydrate protein molecules found in most foods. According to D'Adamo, certain lectins are incompatible with certain blood types. This incompatibility allegedly causes the lectin to attract and clump red blood cells, a process known as agglutination. So when you eat a food containing protein lectins that are incompatible with your blood type antigen, the lectins target organs and begin to agglutinate blood cells in that area. According to D'Adamo, lectin-caused agglutination is the primary cause of many common health complaints. For example, the lectin protein found in milk is not beneficial to blood Type A as it cannot be digested thus causing health problems.

Though the diet wasn't designed for weight-loss per se, D'Adamo claims that weight loss is a natural side effect of the body's restoration, which is prompted by following the appropriate blood type diet. D'Adamo claims that lectin activity of certain foods may slow down the rate of metabolism, not efficiently burning calories. In addition, he says that incompatible lectins interfere with the production of insulin and upset the body's hormonal balance, which in turn causes weight gain.

How it Works

The menus vary greatly, depending upon your blood type. D'Adamo has tested most common foods for blood-type reactions. He organized the results of this testing into food categories that allow people to avoid eating foods containing lectins that are incompatible with their blood type.

The Blood Type diet divides foods into 16 categories:

1. Meats and poultry
2. Seafood
3. Dairy and eggs
4. Oils and fats
5. Nuts and seeds
6. Beans and legumes
7. Cereals
8. Breads and muffins
9. Grains and pasta
10. Vegetables
11. Fruit
12. Juices and fluids
13. Spices
14. Condiments
15. Herbal teas
16. Miscellaneous beverages

Foods in these categories are then broken down into three groups—highly beneficial, neutral, or avoid— according to each of the four blood types.

Here is a summary of recommendations for various blood types by D'Adamo:

Type O

Type O is claimed to be the "original" blood type—the one that everyone had during the Paleolithic era between 50,000 BC and 25,000 BC. The Paleolithic diet was high in meat and was also at a time when few, if any, grain foods were available. Therefore, D'Adamo advocates that Type O people eat a lot of meat, no wheat, and little, if any, other grains. Because early people usually had to be very active (e.g., through the need to hunt animals) he also believes that people with Type O should engage in vigorous aerobic exercise.

Type O, D'Adamo says, is associated with high levels of stomach acid and cholesterol-splitting intestinal enzymes, and can easily metabolize animal protein. It has a greater incidence of blood clotting disorders, as well as gastric ulcer and inflammatory diseases. This blood group should avoid grains, particularly wheat and corn.

Type A

Type A blood type emerged between 25,000 BC and 15,000 BC, a necessary adaptation to a more agrarian lifestyle. As a result, D'Adamo believes that Type A people should eat plenty of grains and other high-carbohydrate foods. Because agriculture does not involve a high level of aerobic exercise, he suggests that Type A people should engage only in "light activity, such as golf and yoga".

Type A secretes smaller amounts of stomach acid and is primarily associated with vegetarian protein. Type A people flourishes on a high-fiber, complex carbohydrate diet, with foods such as tofu, legumes, and beans. They have a high rate of diabetes, heart diseases, and certain cancers, and should avoid dairy and meat.

Type B

Type B blood according to D'Adamo, appeared 10,000 to 15,000 years ago as a result of migration and possible mutation of Type A. Type B people "should have the most varied diet of all the blood types, including meat." D'Adamo also believes that Type B is "the only blood type that does well with dairy products." The forms of exercise that D'Adamo suggests for Type B are "moderate swimming or walking."

Type B is best suited to an omnivorous diet with protein sources from fish and dairy. They have a high incidence of urinary tract diseases such as kidney and bladder infections. They should avoid foods containing corn, chicken, buckwheat, and peanuts.

Type AB

The most recent blood group, according to D'Adamo, is Type AB, which he states did not come into existence until about 1,000 years ago. People with the AB blood type can supposedly eat a reasonably varied diet (but evidently should not consume much in the way of dairy products) and should take part in "calming exercises and relaxation techniques."

Type AB does well with vegetarian protein, dairy, and seafood. They are prone to heart disease, cancer and anemia, and should avoid red meat, corn, buckwheat, and certain beans.

Advantages

- The Blood Type Diet aids in the fight against life-threatening diseases such as cancer, cardiovascular disease, diabetes, and liver failure.
- If you like following a set list of foods that you can and cannot eat this diet may be for you, since there are specific guidelines given for foods, amounts, and timing of meals.
- D'Adamo believes that this diet restores the body's natural genetic rhythm to achieve health and vitality.

- The diet encourages anti-aging and natural body weight maintenance.

Disadvantages

- The Blood Type Diet is unrealistic if members of one family have different blood types, requiring them to each follow a completely different diet.
- Each plan unnecessarily eliminates specific groups of foods, which can result in nutrient deficiency.
- Critics caution that people with Type O blood may increase their risk of heart disease by adhering to D'Adamo's Type O diet recommendations.
- D'Adamo barely addresses exercise, which is a critical component of any weight-loss program. He mainly discusses exercise as a way to reduce stress, not lose weight.

Summary

Nutritionists generally agree that some individuals may have unique eating needs, but basing what you eat on blood type is ridiculous. Nutritionists maintain our basic nutrition needs are the same whether we're A positive, B negative, or any other type.

Nutrition experts argue that D'Adamo's theory about lectins lacks solid scientific support. They point out that the research that has been done on lectins has been performed mostly in test tubes. Furthermore, many food lectins are destroyed by cooking and/or digestive enzymes, so many critics argue that the number of lectins absorbed intact through the digestive system is minimal.

Other critics point out that D'Adamo's emphasis on the ABO blood-typing system is somewhat arbitrary. Medical experts have pointed out that ABO blood typing is only one of many different blood-typing methods, and to date more than 30 unique markers have been identified in the red blood cells. Consequently, if D'Adamo had based his diet on a different marker, his diet recommendations may have been very different.

Of equal concern is his advice that only people with a certain blood type should engage in vigorous physical activity. Being physically active is of the utmost importance to everyone, regardless of blood type.

Although most critics concede that the Blood Type Diet produces weight loss in some people, they argue that this diet is merely a calorie-restricted diet. As with any other low calorie diet, weight loss is likely to occur.

6

Body for Life Diet

Overview

The Body for Life Diet, by Bill Phillips, is a diet and fitness program for those that want to change the shape and fitness of their body. Protein is a major part of this diet, as are complex carbohydrates. It is designed to give you lots of energy. So it has a fair amount of calories as well. The program encourages the use of supplements, shakes, bars, and other highly priced items. People on the diet should experience gradual, healthy weight loss.

The Body for Life Diet is intended to be a lifestyle change. The calories are low enough for overweight people to lose weight, but high enough for an average adult to maintain a reasonable weight. When you reach your desired weight, you should maintain your new eating habits.

How it Works

The Body for Life Diet is a long and extended plan that spreads over 12 weeks. The pattern of eating on Body for Life is six meals a day, six days a week. The diet encourages dieters to count portions of food rather than calories. For each meal, dieters choose one of 18 protein options along with a carbohydrate. Milk and egg products are essential to this diet, as they provide lots of protein. Some people may even invest in protein supplements to make sure they get enough protein. Chicken is usually eaten throughout the day, as it is high in protein and low in fat. Vegetables are also an integral part of the Body for Life Diet. The meals are small in portion size and low in calories, but eating six times a day lessens the hunger pains and reduces the possibility of eating junk foods. One day a week, you are allowed to indulge in your favorite foods.

Another important component in the Body for Life eating plan is the Myoplex formula designed and distributed by Experimental and Applied Sciences, a company owned by Phillips.

You must be willing to exercise regularly in order to benefit from the Body for Life Diet. It is recommended you perform vigorous cardiovascular exercises three times a week, for 20 minutes each session. The other three days you should lift weights (for about 45 minutes per session). Building muscle causes your metabolism to increase, in addition to giving you a leaner and firmer physique. The workouts are suitable for people who want to exercise at home.

Advantages

- The Body for Life Diet claims you get the body you want in 12 weeks.
- It is an excellent curriculum for people wanting to lose weight, or people with ideal weight but wanting to lead a healthier lifestyle.
- The dieter gets one day off each week to indulge in favorite foods.
- The dieter has the option of eating convenient shakes/bars for some of the meals.
- The program gets high marks for motivation.

Disadvantages

- The Body for Life Diet plan lacks specific details of the program.
- The diet is overly strict, and the foods on the authorized list have no special qualities that help with weight loss.
- The supplements, shakes, and bars are expensive.
- You must exercise intensively, six days each week.
- The diet is too rigid and intensive to really be a plan "for life."
- Eating six times a day on a schedule is a problem for most people.
- Non-vegetarian dieters can get their share of proteins, but vegetarian dieters may have problems in meeting their protein needs.

Summary

The Body for Life Diet is good in that encourages a strenuous exercise program, since many diets fail to emphasize the importance in exercising.

Cardiovascular exercises and weight lifting are of the utmost importance to make the Body for Life Diet a success. However, as with all high-protein, low-carbohydrate diets the theories of weight loss remain unproven, and most experts agree they can result in a host of problems, particularly for the large segment of the population that is at risk for heart disease. What's more, these diets don't permit a high intake of fruits and vegetables, in spite of numerous documented health benefits from these foods. In addition, statistics show that dieters who use prepackaged foods fail to learn to make healthy food selections or eat sensible meals and are often at the greatest risk of regaining weight after the program ends.

7

Cabbage Soup Diet

Overview

The Cabbage Soup Diet is based on eating a fat-burning soup that contains negligible calories. The diet promises rapid weight loss by eating as much cabbage soup as you want each day, which should sound appealing to dieters. The recipe for the soup varies slightly, but includes a variety of low-calorie vegetables such as cabbage, onions, and tomatoes, flavored with bouillon, onion soup mix, and tomato juice. While there are no "magical" ingredients in the soup, advocates claim it's a combination of the "superfoods" in the rest of the diet that make the weight disappear. A running myth suggests that this diet originated at any number of hospitals, but thus far no medical facilities have claimed it as their own.

How it Works

Although there are many versions of the Cabbage Soup Diet, typically it's structured to run seven days and then be abandoned for at least two weeks before going back on the diet. The periodic break from the diet is designed to replenish your body's nutrient needs and develop good eating practices. Dieters are encouraged to eat as much cabbage soup as they want and drink seven to eight glasses of water a day. Each day of the seven-day program specific foods must be eaten, including potatoes, fruit juice, and many vegetables. On one day, beef is eaten.

The diet works on the principle that it is low in calories. By giving you guidelines of certain foods to eat on specific days, it is designed to keep the calorie and fat content as low as possible without sacrificing vital nutrients. The working agents are antioxidants and phytochemicals, which work to rid the body of toxins.

The following seven-day meal plan is one version of the Cabbage Soup Diet.

Day One

Eat as much soup as you want, but eat only fruits (no bananas), and drink only unsweetened tea, black coffee, cranberry juice, and water.

Day Two

Eat as much soup as you want but no fruit. Eat raw or cooked leafy green vegetables, but avoid beans, peas, and corn. You can eat a baked potato with butter at dinner.

Day Three

Each as much cabbage soup as you want. You can also eat as much fruit and vegetables as you want, but no baked potatoes.

Day Four

Eat as many as eight bananas and drink as many glasses of skim milk as you would like on this day, along with as much cabbage soup as you want. This day is supposed to lessen your desire for sweets.

Day Five

You may eat as much as 10 to 20 ounces of beef (300–500g) and up to six fresh tomatoes. Drink at least six to eight glasses of water this day to wash the uric acid from your body. Eat cabbage soup at least once this day. You may eat broiled or baked chicken (skinless) or fish instead of beef.

Day Six

Eat beef and vegetables this day. You can even have two or three steaks if you like, with fresh vegetables or salad but no baked potatoes. Eat cabbage soup at least once this day.

Day Seven

Eat all the brown rice and vegetables, and drink all the unsweetened fruit juices you want. Be sure to eat cabbage soup at least once this day. No bread, alcohol, or carbonated beverages—not even diet soda—is allowed.

Advantages

- The Cabbage Soup Diet is affordable and a good break from junk food.
- You'll lose weight quickly and can eat as much as you want of the prescribed foods.
- Vegetables are an important part of all healthy diets.
- Homemade soup is a good slimming food (although any vegetable soup will do) and is reasonably filling.

Disadvantages

- The Cabbage Soup Diet severely restricts your food varieties each day.
- Many people who have tried this diet report feeling light-headed and weak, and notice a decrease in the ability to concentrate.
- The diet is too low in complex carbohydrates, protein, vitamins, and minerals to continue for an extended period of time.
- The weight that you lose through the Cabbage Soup Diet is mostly water, not fat, which means you'll easily gain it back.
- Finally, it doesn't help you to change your eating habits, which is the number one secret of permanent weight loss.

Summary

The general consensus is that the Cabbage Soup Diet is effective in temporary and quick weight loss, but is not effective for long-term weight loss. The obvious criticism of the Cabbage Soup Diet is that it is unbalanced and not a nutritionally sound plan. A diet that focuses on so few foods can't possibly provide all the nutrients you need. In fact, it lacks sufficient quantities of everything from fiber to protein to calcium. However, since the diet is only supposed to be followed for seven days, this shouldn't cause people in good health any long-term problems. People that have special dietary needs, including diabetics, should definitely consult a doctor before starting the Cabbage Soup Diet.

8

Carbohydrate Addict's Diet

Overview

The Carbohydrate Addict's Diet, according to Rachael Heller, M.D., and Richard Heller, M.D., is based on a single theory: many overweight people are "carbohydrate addicts." They define carbohydrate addiction as a compelling hunger, craving, or desire for carbohydrate-rich foods or an escalating, recurring need or drive for starches, snack foods, junk food, or sweets. The Hellers maintain that eating carbohydrates for some people is like doing drugs, and they have devised a diet plan that greatly restricts carbohydrate intake, distributing it in measured amounts at a single meal. Carbohydrate addiction, they say, is not a matter of will power; it is a matter of biology, pure and simple.

According to the Hellers, overproduction of insulin is what triggers hunger and drives the carbohydrate addicts to crave more carbohydrates throughout the day. Eating too many carbohydrates, they say, causes a spike in insulin production, which triggers carbohydrate cravings. This drives you to eat even more carbohydrates, which creates a never-ending cycle of craving, over-consumption of carbohydrates, and overproduction of insulin. An over-indulgence in carbohydrate-rich foods, then, leads to weight gain and out-of-control eating.

The Heller's report that insulin is best managed by simply limiting carbohydrates during most of the day, especially eliminating foods that contain refined carbohydrates, such as sugar and flour. They say that the entire chain of metabolic events is altered with a low-carbohydrate diet: less insulin is released, less fat is stored, and more fat is burned up. Because the body is releasing less insulin, the brain regulates the appetite better with a release of serotonin, a biochemical that gives that nice, complete feeling of satiety.

They recommend you lose no more than 1% of your weight per week. For instance, a person who weighs 200 pounds would aim to lose no more than two-pounds per week, while a person who weighs 150 pounds should only lose 1.5 pounds per week at the most.

How it Works

Though the Hellers' plan is basically a low-carbohydrate diet, it doesn't restrict carbohydrates to the extent that the Atkins Diet does. The Carbohydrate Addict's Diet is divided into three kinds of meals: the Reward Meal, and two carbohydrate-restricted meals known as the Complementary Meal, and the Complementary Snack.

With the Reward Meal you can eat any food you want within a one-hour time period in any quantity, but your plate must be balanced with 1/3 proteins, 1/3 low-carbohydrate vegetables, and 1/3 rich carbohydrates (including desserts). The catch is that if you want second helpings, you have to dish up the same one-third, one-third, one-third distribution on your plate—and eat everything. Part of the reason people can adhere to this diet long-term is that they know, every day, if they have a craving they can satisfy it at the Reward Meal. The Hellers recommend eating complex carbohydrates such as pasta, bread, and potatoes. Sugar is not on the menu. They also recommend eating low-fat most of the time, but allow you to give in to your cravings when you want. With the Reward Meal, nothing is off limits. The Reward Meal can be breakfast, lunch, or dinner.

By limiting the Reward Meal to 60 minutes a day, insulin is kept under control even when a dieter is seriously over-indulging. After a full hour of indulgence you take a 23-hour respite until the next evening's one-hour binge.

The Complementary Meal, on the other hand, consists of one serving (three to four ounces) of meat, fish, or fowl or two ounces of cheese, plus roughly 2 cups of vegetables or salad. Some of the foods not allowed are fruits, broccoli, milk, and yogurt.

While on the diet, you drink plenty of water and are allowed to drink an unlimited amount of sugar-free drinks such as diet sodas, unsweetened tea, seltzer, and black coffee. Only one cup of coffee with cream is allowed, due to the carbohydrate content. Milk, fruit juices, and sugary drinks should be saved for your Reward Meal.

The Hellers recommend that you weight yourself every day. Write down the numbers, average your weight each week, and make changes according to how your weekly average weight compares to the goal weight range that you've set for yourself.

Advantages

- The Carbohydrate Addict's Diet can be used with healthy food choices.
- Helps control your cravings for carbohydrates.

Disadvantages

- The Carbohydrate Addict's Diet seems to have an inadequate nutritional balance.
- The diet does not offer a long-term solution to weight control.
- The diet relies heavily on protein (meat).
- It is easy to make bad food choices at the Reward Meal.
- There is no major emphasis on exercise.
- The lack of concentration that is attributed to overindulging on carbohydrates is actually a symptom of not getting enough carbohydrates. That's because glucose, the sugar the body manufactures from the carbohydrates you eat, is the brain's primary fuel.

Summary

In a nutshell, the Carbohydrate Addict's Diet, though not as extreme as the Atkins Diet, is a low-carbohydrate, high-fat, high protein diet plan, which is not currently recommended by health or dietary organizations. All high-protein, low-carbohydrate plans put the dieter at risk of loss of vitamin B, calcium, and potassium, resulting from lack of carbohydrates in the diet, and risk of coronary heart disease from eating more high-protein foods that are also high in fat.

Nutrition experts don't agree with the Hellers' claim that most overweight people are "carbohydrate addicts." It is well known that many individuals have abnormally high insulin levels and insulin resistance, but this is a part of the medical condition known as the metabolic syndrome, which has a variety of causes—notably obesity itself. Carbohydrate addiction has never been shown to be among the causes.

They have also noted the Hellers' premise that "insulin makes you fat" is unsupported. In fact, researchers have actually found that managing insulin levels does not help you lose weight. However, the reverse has been proved to be true: Losing weight can help control insulin levels.

Like the Atkins Diet and other low-carbohydrate diets, the Hellers' plan is likely to result in weight loss, at least in the beginning. But restricting carbohydrates is not a real-life situation, and it's one that few people would be able to maintain for a lifetime.

9

Caveman Diet

Overview

The Caveman Diet, or Paleolithic Diet is modeled after what our ancient ancestors supposedly ate in prehistoric times, such as fruits, nuts, vegetables, berries, and lean meats. It places a lot of emphasis on protein and takes a step away from cultivated products such as rice and bread. This diet claims that weight loss is best achieved by eating a diet high in protein, with up to 30% of the diet consisting of meat. Although the diet places a lot of emphasis on meat, the wild game eaten in Paleolithic times had far less fat than today's domestically produced meat, and mirrors what's recommended today to lower the risk of heart disease.

How it Works

Although there are many versions of the Caveman Diet, one plan recommends the following meal plan.

Breakfast — a grapefruit and a glass of orange juice

Lunch — a tossed salad and all of the nuts you want to eat

Snacks — as many apples as you desire

Dinner — all the chicken you care to eat, along with two servings of vegetables

Advantages

- The Caveman Diet, being rich in fruits and vegetables, is rich in antioxidants, which have been shown to lower the risk of cancer and heart disease.
- Not eating processed food products reduces the amount of fat, salt, sugar, and chemicals in ones diet, thus leading to a healthier lifestyle.

Disadvantages

- Since the Caveman Diet is very low in carbohydrates, it can also make people feel very tired and weak.
- Cutting dairy and grains out of your diet can result in calcium and vitamin D deficiencies, as well as deficiencies in vitamin B.

Summary

Many aspects of the Caveman Diet are appealing, including the eating of leafy vegetables, fruits, and lean meats, and keeping processed foods to a minimum. However, many nutritionists believe that although lean cuts of meat are fine, the diet is still too high in protein. Also, too much emphasis is on meat for protein and not on other food sources like soy, dairy foods, nuts, and beans. This diet tends to lead to an unhealthy amount of fat consumption and is similar to many of the high protein/low carbohydrate diets today, such as the Atkins Diet, the Zone Diet, and the South Beach Diet.

10

Chicken Soup Diet

Overview

The Chicken Soup Diet is based on eating chicken soup and is basically a calorie-reduction diet plan, which involves losing weight by sharply reducing the number of calories one consumes in a day. This diet plan involves eating much less food and a lot more chicken soup.

How it Works

The Chicken Soup Diet is a very simple diet plan that lasts for one week. You are allowed to eat as much chicken soup as you want during the day, other than for breakfast (see breakfast choices listed below). To get a good nutritional balance from the Chicken Soup Diet you should have a different breakfast every day of the week.

The actual recipe for the chicken soup is quite simple and includes vegetables such as celery, carrots, and broccoli. The other ingredients are quite common, such as chicken and various types of seasonings.

The five breakfast choices for you are:

Breakfast 1
- 1 cup vanilla nonfat yogurt combined with ½ cup chopped fruit salad and sprinkled with wheat germ.

Breakfast 2
- 1 cup ricotta cheese combined with ½ teaspoon of sugar and a dash of cinnamon.
- 2 pieces white-grain bread, toasted
- 3 dried figs

Breakfast 3
- 1-½ cups Total cereal

- ½ cup nonfat milk
- ½ cup calcium enriched orange juice

Breakfast 4

- ½ cup prune juice
- 1 small whole-wheat bagel, topped with 1 ounce of fat-free melted cheddar cheese.

Breakfast 5

- 1-½ cups cooked Wheatena cereal
- ½ cup nonfat milk

Advantages

- The Chicken Soup Diet is very simple to follow, in that all you need to do is eat soup.
- Dieters have lost weight on this diet due to the severe reduction in calories.
- Chicken soup has anti-inflammatory properties, which explains why it soothes sore throats and eases the misery of colds and flu.
- Chicken soup is very healthy to eat.

Disadvantages

- Although some people may truly love chicken soup, it's doubtful that they would want to build their entire eating plans on the Chicken Soup Diet.
- Most dieters find this diet very boring after a week, given the limited choice of food groups.

Summary

If you have a very small amount of weight to lose, or if you want to jump-start a longer-term calorie reduction diet plan, then utilizing the Chicken Soup Diet for a short-term (seven days) might be plausible. The severe reduction in calories will probably help drop some immediate weight, but staying on the diet past seven days is not a good plan. True chicken soup lovers may be able to do this for a week.

11

Curves Diet

Overview

The Curves Diet plan is exclusive to the Curves International Centers franchise, a chain of fitness centers founded by CEO Gary Heavin. The diet as written about in *Curves: Permanent Results without Permanent Dieting*, authored by Gary Heavin and Carol Colman, offers two separate diet strategies: the Low-Carbohydrate Plan, which is a high-protein, low-carbohydrate diet that is not as stringent as the Atkins Diet Plan, and the Low-Calorie Plan, a 1,200-calorie-a-day diet that allows for slightly more carbohydrates but stresses lowering simple carbohydrates in the daily diet.

The Curves Diet teaches portion sizes and emphasizes that nutrition and physical activity are equally important in managing weight and health.

How it Works

The Curve Diet is a three-phase program that offers two plans to choose from—the Low-Carbohydrate Plan and the Low-Calorie Plan. A simple quiz will help you in selecting the right meal plan. For both plans, most carbohydrates are off limits, although carbohydrates are more restricted on the Low-Carbohydrate Plan.

In Phase 1 of the Low-Carbohydrate Plan, which lasts two weeks, carbohydrates are restricted to 20 grams a day to induce rapid weight loss. You can eat unlimited amounts of protein, including Curves' protein shakes, and unlimited amounts of free foods (most vegetables and leafy greens). (The diet allows other types of protein shakes so you are not stuck buying their products.) In Phase 2 you increase carbohydrates to 60 grams a day until you reach your goal weight. Phase 3 is the Metabolic Tune-Up where you eat normally and track your weight over a month to determine your high weight and your low weight.

There's also an exercise program, preferably at a Curves gym, to complement the diet, and vitamin and mineral supplements are recommended.

Advantages

- Weight loss with the Curves Diet can be as much as six to 10 pounds in the first two weeks, followed by one to two pounds a week thereafter.

- If you are a sedentary person who has never exercised or made an effort to eat right, this program will work simply because you are doing something you have never done before.

- The Curves workout is also a great option if you want a comfortable, no frills, time-efficient, weight-loss program.

Disadvantages

- Most Americans already eat more protein than their bodies need, and eating too much protein can increase health risks. High-protein animal foods are usually also high in saturated fat and eating large amounts of high-fat foods for a sustained period raises the risk of coronary heart disease, diabetes, stroke, and several types of cancer.

- People who can't use excess protein effectively may be at higher risk of kidney and liver disorders, and osteoporosis.

- High-protein diets don't provide some essential vitamins, minerals, fiber, or some other nutritional elements.

- There are numerous metabolic and health risks associated with ketosis, including fatigue in late afternoon, hypotension (too-low blood pressure), headaches, constipation, diarrhea, thinning hair, dry skin, altered breath, and muscle cramps.

Summary

Nutritionists like that it teaches portion sizes and emphasizes that nutrition and physical activity is part of the diet program, but have problems with the plans, especially the Low-Carbohydrate Plan, because they limit healthy foods such as fruit and whole grains. Nutritionists also have problems with the Curves Diet because it claims that you can eat unlimited amounts of protein and still lose weight if you cut back on starchy and sugary carbohydrates. This isn't true since any excess calories above the body's needs, including protein, are stored as fat. Simply stated, if you eat too many calories, you will gain weight.

The Curves Diet goes against mainstream nutritional recommendations when it says you can go off the diet when you reach your desired weight and that it shouldn't become a way of life. Nutritionists say the key to long-term weight loss is adopting real-life strategies for healthy eating and exercise habits that you can maintain over a lifetime. Going on and off a diet can lead to rebound binge eating and to gaining back more weight than was lost.

Regardless of the plan you follow, the Curves Diet is effectively a low-carbohydrate diet that is low in calories, which explains its results in weight loss.

12

Detox Diet

Overview

The basic premise behind the Detox Diet is to purify the body by temporarily fasting and giving up certain kinds of foods that are thought to contain toxins. Supporters of the diet claim our bodies are continually overloaded with toxins from, for example, pollution, cigarette smoke, pesticides, a poor diet, food additives, alcohol, and caffeine. As these toxins build up in our digestive, lymph, and gastrointestinal systems, as well as in our skin and hair, any number of health problems can occur, including weight gain, cellulite, headaches, dull skin, bloating, fatigue, lowered immunity, aches and pains, and a general lack of well-being. The process of detoxing involves removing toxins from the body.

While detoxification diets are varied and numerous, in their purest form they involve some fasting and then gradually reintroducing certain foods into the diet. The foods allowed and banned can vary widely among the different detox diets, but generally fruit, vegetables, beans, nuts, seeds, herbal teas, and massive amounts of water are allowed. In contrast, wheat, dairy, meat, fish, eggs, caffeine, alcohol, salt, sugar, and processed foods usually are banned. The recommended duration of this regime also varies, but it may be followed for a minimum of three days, or up to three weeks.

Many of these diets also encourage as part of the purification process a colonic irrigation, otherwise known as an enema (flushing out the rectum and colon using water), which is designed to "clean out" your colon. Still others recommend that you take herbal supplements to help the "purification" process.

How it Works

As mentioned, there are many different variations of the Detox Diet. One 30-day Detox Diet regime requires fasting for first three days drinking only purified water with half a lemon squeezed into it. Instead of water, you can drink freshly made fruit and vegetable juices. During these three days you should keep activity to a minimum and not venture into any extreme climates. Following the three-day fast for the next seven days you must eat only one type of fruit (e.g., melons, citrus, etc.) for each meal. For example, for breakfast you can eat only certain types of melons such as watermelon or cantaloupe. For lunch you might just eat oranges or grapefruit. For an afternoon snack you must drink a glass of fresh carrot juice, and for dinner it's the same story: only eat one type of fruit. During this seven-day period you can eat as much fruit as you want until the hunger is satisfied. For the next 20 days of the diet regime you move to an all raw-food diet as discussed.

Basic Raw-Food Diet

Breakfast

Fresh fruit only such as oranges, kiwis, pineapples, apples, plums, grape-fruits, or any other acidic fruit, can be eaten for breakfast. You can mix the fruits and eat enough to satisfy your hunger.

Lunch

Eat plenty of grapes, pears, bananas, mangoes, and fresh dates, and with this meal eat a head of lettuce, one to two sticks of celery, and a handful of dried raisins or sultanas, or three to four dried figs or 10–12 dried apricots.

Snack

Drink a 12-ounce glass of freshly squeezed carrot juice for a mid-afternoon snack.

Evening

In the evening you can eat a large salad of grated red cabbage, carrots, and beetroot, and chopped up celery, watercress, cucumber, and red or green peppers. A dressing could be made as follows: add two to three tomatoes in the blender, one whole, peeled, large avocado with seed removed, a pinch of marigold bouillon powder, and one teaspoon of cold-pressed linseed oil, flax oil or olive oil. Add just a little water to give the dressing a creamy texture. Blend the ingredients, pour the dressing on your salad, and mix the salad thoroughly. To this salad you can add three ounces of chopped up non-salted nuts and seeds, but no peanuts.

After a month on this diet regime—if you have not cheated in between—you should feel cleaner, fitter, a little slimmer, and more energetic. Remember: No cooked food should be eaten.

Foods to include in a Detox Diet

- Fresh Vegetables - onions, cabbage, peppers, cucumbers, tomatoes, carrots, leeks, artichokes, and salad leaves.
- Fresh Fruits - apples, strawberries, raspberries, cranberries, mangoes, grapes, grapefruits, pineapples, oranges, cantaloupes, and kiwifruit.
- Nuts and Seeds - unsalted nuts (such as walnuts, cashew, brazil nuts, and almonds) and seeds like sunflower, flaxseeds, poppy seeds, and pumpkin seeds.
- Herbs and Spices - chives, mustard, chili, garlic, and ginger.
- Water - If possible, drink only bottled or filtered water. Drink at least eight glasses of water or diluted fruit juice each day.

Foods to Avoid in a Detox Diet

- Red meat, chicken, turkey and any meat products like sausages, burgers, and pate
- Milk, cheese, eggs, butter, margarine, and cream
- Any food that contains wheat, including bread, croissants, cereals, cakes, biscuits, pies, pastry, quiche, battered or breadcrumbed foods, etc.
- Crisp and savory snacks, including salted nuts
- Chocolate, sweets, jam, and sugar
- Processed foods, ready-to-eat meals, ready-made sauces, and takeaways
- Alcohol

- Coffee and tea
- Sauces, pickles, shop-bought salad dressing, and mayonnaise
- Salt

Advantages

- The Detox Diet can prevent and cure diseases, and give you more energy, making you more focused and clear-headed.
- Detox diets will help the system to rid itself of stored toxins and take pressure off your kidneys, liver, bowels, and lymph system.
- Detox diets do encourage some good habits, such as eating more fruit and vegetables, drinking more water and cutting down on junk food and processed foods. Plus they encourage you to cut back on caffeine and alcohol—all of which are good habits.
- Detox diets do help you lose weight, but this is because calorie intakes are usually extremely low. This is because you're cutting out major groups of foods, such as dairy products, meat, and wheat-based foods.

Disadvantages

- Detox diets can be addicting, because there's a certain feeling that comes from going without food or having an enema—almost like the high other people get from nicotine or alcohol.
- The main problem relates to the fact that detox diets can be short on many nutrients, leading to certain deficiencies and lowered immunity. For example, by eliminating dairy products from your diet, it's very hard to meet nutrition needs for calcium, a mineral that's needed for strong bones and teeth. And, in the long term, a deficiency of calcium can lead to osteoporosis—brittle bone disease—in later life.
- The point of the Detox Diet is to purify the body from chronic ailments, and thus it can be quite a hard diet to manage. For starters, you must fast before you can even go on the diet.
- It's not recommended that people with diabetes, low blood sugar, or eating disorders go on a Detox Diet.

- Many of the supplements called for by these diets are actually laxatives, which can cause dehydration, mineral imbalances, and problems with your digestive system.

- If you fast for several days, you may drop pounds, but most of it will be water and some of it may be muscle, which will make you look thin and flabby, rather than tight and toned. Fasting for longer periods can also slow down your metabolism, making it harder to keep the weight off or to lose weight later.

- Detox diets can be especially risky for people who are involved in sports and physical activities that require ample food.

- A problem with many detox diets is that they're tough to follow and it's practically impossible to sustain such a limited diet for a long period of time. That's why detox diets aren't the answer to long-term weight loss.

Summary

Although detox diets may make you feel better, there is no scientific proof that a detox diet will help rid the body of toxins faster, or even if they do, that the elimination of toxins will make you healthier. Of course, it's true that food isn't all pure nutrients, and the average diet will inevitably contain some toxic substances (alcohol, for example). Fortunately, the human body is well equipped to deal with such toxins; they are eliminated or neutralized through the colon, liver, kidneys, lungs, lymph glands, and skin.

The basic misconception of detox diets, however, is that fruits and vegetables are low in toxins, while meat and fish lead to the accumulation of harmful substances in the body. In fact, the opposite is often true; vegetables such as cabbage and onions are high in naturally occurring toxins, while meat and fish often have low levels.

Of course, fruit and vegetables are very important components of a healthy diet, but the idea that you should exist solely on such foods for days on end isn't consistent with the principle of a healthy balanced diet. Your daily diet should contain at least five portions of fruit and vegetables as well as lean meat, carbohydrates, and dairy products.

13

Eat to Live Diet

Overview

The Eat to Live Diet is a nutritional program developed by Dr. Joel Fuhrman, M.D., and is described in detail in his book of the same name. Basically, the idea of the Eat to Live Diet is to eat foods that have a very high nutrition-to-calorie ratio, such as fruits and vegetables, and avoid foods that don't provide much nutrition for the calories they contain. Essentially, the program is a low-calorie vegetarian diet with an emphasis on raw vegetables.

The diet is based on the formula "Health=Nutrients/Calories," which means that when the ratio of nutrients to calories is high, the fat will melt away. The more nutrient-rich food you consume, the more you will be satisfied with fewer calories, and the cravings for fattening foods will disappear.

How it Works

Under Fuhrman's six-week program you can eat an unlimited amount of raw vegetables (including carrots), cooked green vegetables, beans, legumes, sprouts, fresh fruit, eggplant, mushrooms, peppers, onions, and tomatoes. In fact, the goal is to try to eat at least one pound daily of raw vegetables; one pound of cooked, non-starchy vegetables; four servings of fruit; and one cup of beans.

Limits are placed on the consumption of cooked starchy vegetables, whole grains, raw nuts and seeds, avocados, tofu, and ground flaxseed. Cooked starchy vegetables or whole grains are restricted to one cup each day. In this category he includes butternut or acorn squash, corn, potatoes, rice, cooked carrots, sweet potatoes, breads, and cereals.

Most of the fat in this six-week plan comes from raw nuts and seeds, avocados, and ground flaxseed. Fuhrman's prescribed daily maximum amounts are one ounce of raw nuts and seeds, two ounces of avocado, and one tablespoon of ground flaxseed.

All animal products and refined oils are off limits, and refined grain products, such as bread, are not encouraged.

After the initial six-week program, very limited amounts of less-healthy food may be added in (for those who absolutely cannot give them up).

Advantages

- The Eat to Live Diet is good for loosing weight.
- The diet will reverse high blood pressure heart disease and diabetes.
- The diet will help prevent cancer.
- People are purported to live longer while on this diet.

Disadvantages

- The Eat to Live Diet might be considered by some to be monotonous and devoid of taste.
- Some vegetarians may have to supplement the diet with vitamin B12, vitamin D, calcium, zinc, and occasionally riboflavin.
- Vegetarians may have a greater risk of iron deficiency than non-vegetarians.

Summary

The Eat To Live Diet is a balanced vegetarian diet that is not only perfectly healthy but has very real health benefits. Studies continuously show vegetarians have lower incidences of heart disease, diabetes, high blood pressure, and certain forms of cancer than those whose diet is high in protein. More and more evidence is emerging in favor of the health benefits of a cereal- and grain-rich diet.

Typically people following the Eat To Live Diet will lose weight faster than those whose diet is made up of meat. This can be attributed to the fact that most vegetarian diets are comprised mainly of complex carbohydrates. Complex carbohydrates are starchy, fiber-rich foods, and are naturally low in fat.

eDiets Weight Loss Diet

Overview

eDiets.com is an online subscription-based weight loss company that originated with the eDiets Weight Loss Diet, a low-fat weight loss plan based on the recommendations of the American Dietetic Association and the U.S. Department of Agriculture's Food Guide Pyramid. eDiets.com has since expanded its offerings to alternative nutrition plans including the Atkins Diet, The Zone Diet, Dr. Phil's Shape Up Diet, vegetarian, low-cholesterol, and many others.

A subscription or membership includes weekly meal plans, a virtual fitness trainer, online support and counseling from nutritionists, member chat rooms, and 24/7 access to a wealth of information regarding nutrition, exercise and motivation.

How it Works

The eDiets Weight Loss Diet is a highly personalized and customized diet plan meant to take into account every individual's different needs and goals. Whatever a person's tastes, preferences, and dietary needs, this plan may be customized accordingly. Also, the plan may be changed at any time and is noted for its wide variety and good balance. You may also obtain access to a variety of other services, like forums and counseling, although some of those weight loss services cost extra.

The eDiet Weight Loss Diet is based on structured meal plans, accessible only online at their website, using typical grocery store package foods and recipes with minimal substitutions. Meals vary according to each individual's needs and desires. Healthy choices are always encouraged, but an attempt is made to include a person's favorite foods in the diet. Consequently, this diet is not so much about what one cannot eat as it is about what one can eat, and how to make healthier choices from the foods a person is already eating. For example, if fast foods are the only option one day, this plan can suggest ways to make the meal as healthy as possible.

This plan focuses more on food than it does on exercise.

Advantages

- The eDiets Weight Loss Diet has structured meal plans that are simple to follow because the thinking is done for you, which can be helpful in the short term.
- The diet is regarded as a good plan for losing and controlling weight.
- There are no meetings to attend while on this diet.

Disadvantages

- The eDiets Weight Loss Diet rigid meal plans can get boring quickly and many may find it hard to make food choices outside of the meal plan structure.
- The cost is not unreasonable, but at around $250 per year, if you want support, it can be expensive.
- Pay attention to the small print and additional offerings that more-or-less require purchases in the future, such as food, supplements, energy bars, shakes, etc.

Summary

The eDiets Weight Loss Diet is a healthy, low-fat regimen based upon healthy guidelines and is well balanced, according to most nutritionists. The problem comes when dieters opt out of the eDiets plan and choose some of the other popular regimens the site now offers, such as Atkins or The Zone—plans that may provide unhealthy levels of saturated fat or far too few calories to be adequate.

15

Fat Flush Diet

Overview

The Fat Flush Diet developed by Ann Louise Gittleman is a program that targets cleansing of the liver based on eating a combination of healthy essential fats, balanced proteins and good carbohydrates. Gittleman believes this detoxifying process boosts the liver's ability to function at its highest level while accelerating weight loss and improving your health. She maintains the Fat Flush Diet is the only diet program that can successfully break through the stubborn weight loss plateau every dieter faces, and "flush out" stubborn fat, while retaining crucial nutrients.

The Fat Flush process also sets off a domino effect of health benefits, including:

- increasing your metabolism
- giving you more energy
- helping you get a more restful night's sleep
- stabilizing your moods

How it Works

The Fat Flush Diet is a progressing diet plan that transitions from a very strict plan into a trained and later conventional diet in its final phases. The Fat Flush Diet can be subdivided into three phases:

- Phase 1: The Two-Week Fat Flush
- Phase 2: The Ongoing Fat Flush
- Phase 3: The Lifestyle Eating Plan.

Phase 1: The Two-Week Fat Flush

Phase 1, the Two-Week Fat Flush phase, is the purification phase, cleansing the liver in order to achieve effective weight loss. This is the strictest phase of the plan with a calorie restriction of from 1,100 to 1,200 calories per day and a limited choice of food designed to jumpstart weight loss. The intention here is to "lose bloat," which refers to reducing water retention as well as some fat loss. This phase can be extended beyond the first two weeks.

In this phase you are not allowed to eat margarine, alcohol, sugar, oils or fats (except flaxseed oil), grains, bread, cereal, starchy vegetables (e.g., beans, potatoes, corn, parsnips, carrots, peas, pumpkins), or dairy products. Even herbs and spices are restricted to a small list.

Phase 2: The Ongoing Fat Flush

Phase 2, the Ongoing Fat Flush phase, allows slightly more calories and carbohydrates. This phase is designed for those individuals who have additional weight to lose but who also want to pursue a more moderate cleansing program and enjoy more variety in food choices while still losing weight. The idea is to continue on with the program until the desired weight loss is achieved with a calorie restriction of between 1,200 to 1,500 calories per day.

Phase 3: The Lifestyle Eating Plan

Phase 3, the Lifestyle Eating Plan, is really the Fat Flush maintenance program for lifetime weight control. This phase offers over 1,500 calories daily, providing a basic lifelong eating program designed to increase your vitality and well-being for life. During this phase some starchy carbohydrates are gradually re-introduced, along with gluten-free grains, and some dairy products. At this stage of the diet program your daily percentages of nutrients typically amount to 40% carbohydrates, 30% protein, and 30% fat. As in Phase 2, you will add these foods one at a time to make sure that you are tolerating the new additions without any allergic symptoms. This is the final phase of the Fat Flush Diet plan where the human body is effectively trained for the Fat Flush process, enhancing weight control and keeping healthy at the same time.

The program contains a significant exercise component varying anywhere from 20 to 40 minutes of exercise per day, depending on the phase. Typically, the exercise is low-impact (walking). Strength training (lifting weights) is also recommended twice a week. In addition, the diet plan recommends eight hours of sleep a night.

Advantages

- The Fat Flush Diet helps promotes exercise.
- The Fat Flush program has all the elements of a good and healthy weight loss program.
- Many people like the liver-cleansing properties of the plan.
- Meals are planned for you, and if you don't want what is on the menu, you can make a similar ingredient substitute.
- It emphasizes a wide variety of antioxidant-rich vegetables at each meal. Vegetables are an excellent source of phytochemicals, which can protect against some cancers and heart disease.
- Flaxseeds are a good source of essential fats called omega-3 fats, which have been shown to be protective against heart disease.
- On the whole, this plan is quite easy to follow and there aren't any difficult calculations to be done.

Disadvantages

- The Fat Flush Diet one-size-fits-all approach will never suit everyone. Eight hours of sleep a night may be excellent for some people, but given the recommended exercise program, eight hours of sleep may not be enough for other people.
- Protein-rich foods are often high in fat and saturated fat, which can increase the risk of heart disease. A dieter will need to choose low-fat versions wherever possible such as pork fillet, chicken breast, or other lean cuts of meat.
- One criticism is that the calorie level in Phase 1 of this diet may be too low for some people (particularly men), and the lower calorie levels could have the effect of slowing down metabolism rather than speeding it up.
- Because starchy carbohydrates are restricted, it's hard to follow this eating plan for a long period of time especially for people who like eating carbohydrates.

- Dairy foods are also restricted in the first phase of the diet. These foods are one of the main sources of calcium for many people and are needed to maintain strong teeth and healthy bones. Long-term deficiency may increase the risk of osteoporosis in later life.

- Dietary supplements are recommended, which makes this an expensive diet plan to follow.

Summary

Although there's nothing wrong with telling people to exercise and get adequate sleep, the Fat Flush Diet plan is unbalanced, with an over-emphasis on protein-rich foods. Eliminating starchy carbohydrates and dairy foods means that you could be missing out on naturally occurring vitamins, minerals, and other nutrients. It's nothing more than just a low-calorie diet.

Also, nutritionists question the whole concept of "fat-flushing"—that the liver needs to be detoxified by eating certain foods to accelerate weight loss. There's no science behind this claim.

16

Fit for Life Diet

Overview

The Fit for Life Diet originated in the 1980s in a book written by Harvey and Marilyn Diamond. Basically it is a food-combining weight-loss diet that has two basic tenets: 1) It's not what you eat but when you eat and how you combine your food that determines weight loss and health. 2) Always eat fruit alone, never with other foods. The Diamonds maintain that following these tenets will lead to weight reduction and increased energy levels. They further claim that the body experiences three digestive cycles during the day: appropriation, which is eating and digesting (noon to 8 p.m.); assimilation, which is absorption and the use of nutrients (8 p.m. to 4 a.m.); and elimination of body wastes (4 a.m. to noon). According to the Fit for Life Diet theory, by eating foods in the right combination at the right times, following these natural cycles, the body can rid itself of toxins and excess weight.

How it Works

According to the Diamonds, combining certain foods is at a meal is undesirable. Any food besides fruits and vegetables is considered a "concentrated food" (having a low water content), and concentrated foods cannot be combined with one another. Fruit must be eaten alone. For example, a typical day's menu would begin with only fruit or fruit juice before noon. For lunch and dinner you can either have a carbohydrate-based meal, which would be grains, beans, and vegetables, or a protein-based meal, which would be protein and vegetables. A fruit snack is allowed after dinner, but only if you wait at least three hours after eating dinner. Fruits are okay during the day because of their high water content, which washes and cleanses the body of toxins. However, if fruit is eaten at the end of a meal, it ferments and causes digestion and weight problems. According to the Diamonds, actually drinking water with a meal can be debilitating.

Eating inappropriate combinations of foods will, they claim, lead to "putre-faction" (that is, rotting) of the food in the intestine, which turns to fat. The greatest mistake, they believe, comes from combining protein and carbohydrate foods such as meat with potatoes, eggs with toast, or bread with cheese. Consequently, for lunch or dinner you can either have a carbohydrate-based meal including grains, beans, and vegetables, or a protein meal with some vegetables.

They also claim that if you eat while ill, the food will putrefy in your intestine. Fasting, they say, is a safe and valuable method of eliminating these putrefied foods from the intestine.

Dairy foods and refined sugar are banned because refining "strips every vestige of life" from the sugar, which leads to putrefaction even when the sugars are not combined with other foods.

Advantages

- The Fit for Life Diet encourages dieters to eat lots of fruits and vegetables.
- You can eat as much of the specific foods you want, since there is never a reason to measure portions or worry about counting calories or grams of fat.
- The Fit for Life Diet leads to better digestion of foods.

Disadvantages

- In reality, the Fit for Life Diet isn't all that simple since you can't eat fruits with other foods, and you must not combine proteins and starches.
- Dieters who are into the meat-potato-vegetable routine are in for some dramatic changes.
- Due to limited food choices, protein, zinc, vitamin D, and vitamin B12 are consumed in insufficient amounts.
- The ban on dairy foods certainly jeopardizes calcium intake, as dairy products account for over 70% of the calcium in the Ameri-

can diet. This is particularly true since there are no indications which vegetables are calcium rich.

- The Diamonds urge dieters to ignore signals that something could be wrong, such as diarrhea, dizziness, or headaches, which they attribute to the body ridding itself of toxins.

- They recommend the diet even if you're pregnant.

Summary

The idea of food combining has been around since the turn of the century, and is relatively outdated. The Fit for Life Diet theories are, for the most part, unsupported by scientific or clinical evidence. For example, the Fit for Life Diet premise that we cannot digest a combination of foods has no scientific validity whatsoever. Nutritionists say the human digestive system has the enzymes and other conditions necessary for digesting and absorbing an extremely wide range of foods, whether eaten in isolation or in combinations. Human beings are naturally omnivorous and we can eat grain foods, vegetables, fruits, meat, fish, and dairy products (among many other foods) and thrive on a huge variety of combinations of foods.

With regard to their advice not to combine foods, it is actually quite difficult to avoid combining proteins with carbohydrates. The Diamonds seem to be unaware that the "carbohydrate foods" bread, potatoes, rice, spaghetti, and legumes (foods such as beans, peas, soy products and lentils) also contain significant quantities of protein. Eating these foods on their own (which they regard as appropriate) constitutes the very act of food-combining that they seem to think will cause indigestion.

Anyone who sticks with the Fit for Life Diet will likely lose weight, not because the food-combining diet rids the body of fat-causing toxins, but rather because it's quite restrictive and low in calories.

17

Food-Combining Diets

Overview

Food-combining diets first came to prominence with the Hay Diet in the 1930s, and have gained popularity in recent years. There are several food-combining diets on the market, such as the popular Fit for Life Diet. Food-combining diets are generally based on the theory that in order to optimize digestion and weight loss, specific foods are to be eaten at certain times and eaten in the following combinations:

- Proteins (beans, nuts, seeds, meat, fish, and poultry) and carbohydrates (grains, pasta, breads, cereal, rice, carrots, etc.) should be eaten at separate meals. However, proteins can be eaten with vegetables and starches can be combined with vegetables.
- Fruits should be eaten alone.
- Dairy products are prohibited, as are some other food products depending on the particular type of diet.

Some versions advocate eating only fruit or fruit juices before noon, and focus on other types of food for the remainder of the day. A typical food-combining diet lasts for five weeks, although some versions are indefinite.

How it Works

Digestive enzymes are secreted in very specific amounts and at very specific times. Different food types require different digestive secretions. Carbohydrate foods require carbohydrate-splitting enzymes, whereas protein foods require protein-splitting enzymes. The rules for food combining are briefly explained below.

1. One major part of this diet is not allowing proteins to mix with carbohydrates. You should allow at least four hours between eating proteins and carbohydrates so as to not mix them.

2. Carbohydrate foods and acid foods should not be eaten at the same meal. For example, do not eat bread, rice, or potatoes with

lemons, limes, oranges, grapefruits, pineapples, tomatoes, or other acidic fruits.

3. Tomatoes should be eaten with leafy vegetables and fat foods, and never combined with carbohydrate foods since the acids in the tomato could interfere with the digestion of carbohydrates.

4. Avoid eating nuts and meat, eggs and meat, cheese and nuts, cheese and eggs, meat and milk, eggs and milk, or nuts and milk at the same meal.

5. Do not eat fats with proteins such as cream, butter, or oil with meat, eggs, cheese, or nuts.

6. Fruits should not be eaten with other foods.

7. Eat only one concentrated carbohydrate food at a meal to avoid overeating at meals.

8. Milk is best when drunk alone.

9. Alcohol is allowed in moderation.

Advantages

- Food-combining diets encourage eating fruits and vegetables.

- A food-combining diet may benefit you for a couple of days, as a type of detox diet.

- Due to the very-low calorie nature of the early stages of the diet and the limits on types of foods allowed, weight loss is virtually assured.

Disadvantages

- Food-combining diets can be difficult and time-consuming to follow. Favorite pairings, such as chicken with potatoes, tofu with rice, soy-milk fruit shakes, beans and rice, and tuna sandwiches are not allowed.

- Lacking firm scientific basis, many food-combining diets provide inadequate vitamins and minerals. Protein and carbohydrates cannot be eaten together, so people have to choose one or the other. As a result, people often consume more carbohydrates than protein, as carbohydrates tend to be more filling and satisfying.

Special care should be taken to ensure adequate intake of protein, calcium, zinc, vitamin D, and vitamin B12.

- Food-combining diets may fall below minimum recommended calorie levels.

Summary

Although food-combining diets have helped a number of people with dietary and weight loss problems, there is no hard scientific evidence to support the theory behind these diets. Nutritionists say the idea that weight loss is more likely if you separate certain foods is completely without foundation. In fact, many health practitioners believe that combining protein and carbohydrates can be beneficial. When protein and fats are combined with carbohydrates, the absorption of carbohydrates is slowed. This helps to maintain stable blood sugar and insulin levels and prevent cravings.

French Diet

Overview

Much has been written in recent years about the French Diet. The French drink lots of wine and eat high-fat foods such as flaky croissants, creamy sauces, red meat, butter and cheese, and decadent pastries, but still stay slim and have less heart disease than Americans.

In fact, despite their rich diet, the French generally are slimmer than Americans. Although no scientific studies are cited, reportedly just 8% of the French qualify as obese, compared to 33% of Americans. As for the widely held idea that the French are thin because they smoke more, it's a myth. An estimated 21% of French women smoke, and 33% of French men, compared with 20% of U.S. women and 25% of men, the American Cancer Society says—not enough of a difference to be statistically different.

The "French paradox"—the perplexing disconnect between France's rich cuisine and slender population—can be explained in part by the smaller portions they eat. While the French eat more fat than Americans, they probably eat fewer total calories, which when compounded over years, can amount to substantial differences in weight.

How it Works

The eating patterns of the French offer significant clues to their healthfulness. For one, like Americans, the French traditionally consume three meals a day. But that's where the similarity ends. The French generally consume 60% of their day's calories before mid afternoon, followed later by a small dinner. For the French, lunch and dinner are the most structured meals, consisting of a starter, such as crudite (raw vegetables), followed by a main course, a salad, the cheese course, and perhaps dessert. Their substantial lunch and dinner often usurps the need for a snack. As a result, snacking is simply not part of the culture. The French believe eating between meals can be a problem and is clearly unhealthy. In the U.S. we typically eat about three high-fat, high-calorie snacks a day.

Meals in France traditionally are regarded as experiences to be savored—sanctimonious time-outs that a snack can otherwise spoil. Food is a life pleasure, and it's meant to be enjoyed. For both lunch and dinner, people tend not to rush if they can help it.

There are some hints and suggestions for adapting to a new way of enjoying food and eating *à la française*.

- Eat three good meals a day.
- Remember that it is quality that counts, not quantity.
- Take smaller bites and finish each completely before taking the next one.
- Eat a wide variety of fresh foods, including plenty of fruits and vegetables, but not a lot at one sitting.
- Eat a certain amount of dairy fat and olive oil with meals.
- Avoid eating processed foods, not faux foods like chips, sodas, Fruit Roll-ups, or cheddar Goldfish.
- Learn to eat slowly—make eating a special time.
- Drink plenty of water.
- Drink a glass of wine with meals.
- Eat dessert—but save room for it by having smaller portions of other courses.
- Walk everywhere, including up and down the stairs

Advantages

- The French Diet has not only been proven to reduce the risk factors for heart disease but will also help prevent and control the ravages of all chronic illnesses including obesity, hypertension, diabetes, cancer, and inflammatory conditions.
- The French Diet is not as restrictive as some of the other diets.

- Not eating processed food products reduces the amount of the amount of fat, salt, sugar, and chemicals in one's diet, thus leading to a healthier lifestyle.
- It is not a weight loss diet, but rather a health plan that will assist your body to reach and maintain its optimal weight.
- The diet promotes daily exercise.

Disadvantages

- Some dieters have complained it was hard to adapt to the French Diet because it differed significantly from their own dietary eating habits.

Summary

Most nutritionists give the French Diet an enthusiastic stamp of approval but believe switching to the French approach to food would take a major change in attitude for most people. Americans often see food as a job or errand that they have to do quickly so they can get back to work, unlike the French who really do love their food. Most nutritionists think Americans could learn a few things from the French when it comes to eating—for one, they aren't obsessed with counting carbohydrates, fat grams, or calories. To them, eating is about enjoying all kinds of foods in moderation. Bon appétit!

19

Get With the Program Diet

Overview

Bob Green's Get With the Program Diet is not a diet, but rather an eating and exercise plan that focuses on getting rid of emotional and haphazard eating while making exercise an important part of followers' lifestyles. Bob Greene is one of the more well-known fitness and weight loss gurus, having made a name for himself as the personal trainer for Oprah Winfrey. The Get With the Program Diet focuses on sensible lifestyle changes that don't require drastic alterations in the types of food followers can and cannot eat. This plan focuses on health, sensible eating choices, and lifestyle decisions intended to be followed throughout one's life.

The initial focus of the program is on exercise in order to raise metabolism, with less focus on calorie counting than on determining why you overeat. Bob Greene refers to this as "emotional eating."

How it Works

Get With the Program Diet stresses healthy eating and eating only when you're hungry. There are not as many noticeable food restrictions as there are with some other diets, mainly because the Get With the Program Diet is not so much a diet as an attempt to change people's attitudes towards food. Haphazard and emotional eating are both strongly discouraged.

This eating plan recommends getting into a routine fitness regimen before trying to reduce calorie intake or change eating habits. Once you start to look and feel better, the guilt of poisoning your body with poor nutrition becomes a powerful controlling factor. This eating plan really focuses on combining both eating and exercising and integrating both to produce a healthy lifestyle.

Advantages

- The Get With the Program Diet helps promote exercise.
- The Get With the Program Diet has all the elements of a good and healthy weight loss program.

Disadvantages

- The Get With the Program Diet portion sizes aren't specified, which means it's possible that dieters, when left to their own devices, could end up overeating.
- The diet requires a major time commitment (one hour a day) for exercise—something that not everyone can commit to.

Summary

Nutritionists say Get With the Program Diet is overall a good balanced diet. If there's one downside to the program, it's that it's heavily slanted toward exercise advice. Anyone who eats when they're stressed, bored, angry or sad should take a look at this diet.

20

G.I. Diet

Overview

The G.I. Diet developed by Rick Gallop, former president of the Heart and Stroke Foundation of Ontario, offers a unique diet program based on the Glycemic Index (GI). The theory behind the diet is that foods with a low GI value slowly release sugar into the blood, providing you with a steady supply of energy. This gives you a more satisfied feeling so that you're less likely to snack. In contrast, foods with a high GI value cause a rapid—but short-lived—rise in blood sugar. This leaves you lacking in energy and feeling hungry within a short time, causing you to eat more food. If this pattern is frequently repeated, you're likely to gain weight as a result of constantly overeating.

Most high-GI foods, such as those made from white flour are heavily processed and the essential nutrients have been stripped away. Conversely, low-GI foods, such as fruits, vegetables, nuts, legumes, whole grains, lean meat/fish, and low-fat dairy are rich in nutrients essential for your good health.

How it Works

With the G.I. Diet, foods are classified according to how quickly they are absorbed into the system, helping you recognize which foods will make you feel fuller for longer. This program is easy to follow, as the G.I. Diet makes all the calculations for you by organizing all the foods in one of three categories: red light foods, which you avoid if you want to lose weight; yellow light foods that can be eaten occasionally; and green light foods that can be eaten as much as you like.

Green light foods are essentially fruits and vegetables. The yellow light foods, such as bananas and steak, can be eaten once in a while and in moderation. And the red light foods, such as pizza, bagels, and bacon, are the ones people should stay away from if they want to lose weight.

The plan recommends eating low-GI foods such as spinach and oranges to keep hunger in check, insulin levels low, and fat at bay. The diet also recommends combining low-GI foods with small portions of low-fat and low-calorie foods, such as high-fiber bread and wild rice, lean protein and fat-free sugar-free yogurt. It is okay to enjoy caffeine-free diet soft drinks and red wine in moderation, skipping regular coffee and sugary soft drinks. Portion sizes should be increased until weight stabilizes at your target body mass index.

Advantages

- The G.I. Diet is not only good for losing weight, but has been found to reduce "bad" LDL cholesterol.
- Unlike the Atkins Diet, which bans most carbohydrates, especially in the early stages, the G.I. diet, actively encourages you to eat many carbohydrates and antioxidant-rich fruits and vegetables.
- The diet is high in fiber, which means you're less likely to become constipated.
- The G.I. Diet also tends to follow healthy eating guidelines and is low in fat, especially saturated fats.
- Following a diet that includes plenty of foods with a low GI value may have a role in helping to prevent or reduce the risk of getting Type 2 diabetes.
- The G.I. Diet is much easier to follow if you are a vegetarian.

Disadvantages

- One of the main limitations of the G.I. Diet is the fact that it's difficult to estimate the GI value of a meal.
- You might experience nutritional deficiencies from not eating higher-GI foods.
- Some foods with a low GI value are also packed with fat and/or salt and contain few nutrients.

Summary

In general, most nutritionists are supportive of the basic principles of the G.I. Diet. The diet generally contains plenty of fruit and vegetables, and recommends eating fewer refined carbohydrates. They do, however, believe that many popular diet authors have taken a controversial nutritional concept—the Glycemic Index—out of the context for which it was intended: as a guideline for diabetics.

Also, critics contend the diet's color-coding system only identifies the effect different foods have on blood sugar levels when they are eaten on their own and, consequently, many believe this is one of the main problems with the G.I. Diet. Basically, when you eat foods together, as in a meal, the GI value of that whole meal is reflected in portion sizes and the individual GI values for each food eaten. As a guideline, the more low-GI foods you include in a meal, the lower the overall GI value for that meal. For instance, mashed potatoes have a high GI value, but if the meal includes pan-seared salmon, a big salad, and steamed broccoli—all of which have low GI values—these foods will minimize the impact on blood sugar levels that come from eating the potatoes.

However, many nutritionists give Gallop credit for keeping the choices on his red-light and green-light lists healthful. The green-light list offers a full menu of low-fat, high-nutrient foods including lean meats, fish, whole grains, fruits, and vegetables. Chocolate-covered peanuts may have a low Glycemic Index, but on the G.I. Diet, candy is a red-light food. Ditto for low-glycemic but fatty meats like bacon and sausage.

21

Grapefruit Diet

Overview

There are many versions of the Grapefruit Diet, but typically the diet calls for eating a few select vegetables, limited protein, plus the all-important serving of grapefruit. This diet claims that grapefruit contains a special fat-burning enzyme that is activated when you eat grapefruit at each meal, along with small amounts of other food.

How it Works

The basis of the Grapefruit Diet is that you eat a half a grapefruit at all three meals. In order to properly follow the grapefruit diet, it is imperative that you eat every meal. Skipping meals may slow down your metabolism and slow down weight loss. The more grapefruit you eat, the more weight you will lose.

This regimented diet does not allow most complex carbohydrates, and doesn't allow for snacking in between meals. However, the consumption of most vegetables is encouraged, and you are allowed to prepare them in generous amounts of butter. It is also recommended that participants drink about eight glasses of water per day.

The grapefruit diet lasts 12 days, but if an individual wants to continue they must take at least two days off before doing so.

Below is a typical meal plan for one day on the Grapefruit Diet

Breakfast:

- One-half grapefruit, or eight ounces unsweetened grapefruit juice
- Two slices bacon
- Two eggs, boiled
- Black coffee (no sugar), or unsweetened tea, if desired

Lunch:

- One-half grapefruit, or eight ounces unsweetened grapefruit juice
- One cup of salad with tomato and low calorie dressing
- Eight ounces lean chicken, tuna, or fish
- Black coffee (no sugar), or unsweetened tea, if desired

Dinner:

- One-half grapefruit, or eight ounces unsweetened grapefruit juice
- Salad: as much as you'd like with dressing of your choice
- Eight ounces of chicken, lean red meat, pork, or fish; use herbs for seasoning
- Black coffee (no sugar), or unsweetened tea, if desired

Advantages

- The Grapefruit Diet produces quick weight loss, primarily due to loss of body water.
- You don't have to count calories.
- Grapefruit has no fat, is low in calories and sodium, and is packed with vitamin C; the pink variety contributes beta-carotene.

Disadvantages

- The Grapefruit Diet is very low in calories.
- It encourages you to drink copious amounts of beverages containing caffeine, making this diet dangerous.
- It's too low in protein, fiber, and several important vitamins and minerals.
- Any diet that relies so much on a single food is too restrictive.
- The Grapefruit Diet is considered monotonous, given the narrow range of foods.
- Needless to say, it doesn't help you to change your eating habits, which is the number one secret to permanent weight loss.

Summary

Although there are compounds in grapefruit that have health-promoting properties, particularly in terms of cancer reduction, there is no scientific basis that grapefruit has a special fat-burning enzyme. Grapefruit is a good food, but so are other healthy foods like vegetables and other fruits. The Grapefruit Diet is effective in losing weight because you are consuming fewer calories than your body needs, grapefruit or no grapefruit.

22

Hamptons Diet

Overview

The Hamptons Diet is a low-carbohydrate diet developed by Dr. Fred Pescatore, former medical director of the Atkins Center. The basic premise of the Hamptons Diet is to eat more vegetables, fish, and omega-3 fatty acids, and to consume most of your fats in the form of monounsaturated fats, a premise shared by the Mediterranean Diet.

Central to the Hamptons Diet is the secret ingredient macadamia nut oil, which Pescatore claims to be "the most monounsaturated oil on the planet." This oil is basically used for everything from salad dressings to marinades and even for cooking. The oils in macadamia are 84% monounsaturated, 3.5% polyunsaturated, and 12.5% saturated. The monounsaturated portion contains oleic fatty acid plus the highest known level of paimitoleic fatty acid, which is also present in beneficial fish oils, and may be nutritionally significant.

Macadamia nuts contain no cholesterol and no trans-fatty acids, and improve the balance between omega-6 and omega-3 fatty acids. This facilitates the body's manufacture of essential fatty acids and eicosanoids (prostaglandins, etc.).

The primary monounsaturated fat that is used in the Mediterranean Diet is olive oil. The traditional Atkins Diet does not distinguish between good fats and bad fats. The Hamptons Diet makes healthy oils a foundation of its nutritional advice.

Emphasis in the diet is on grains and lean proteins such as fish, chicken and fresh vegetables (no fatty steaks like the Atkins) and not all carbohydrates are cut out as with the Atkins Diet. The focus is on the good carbohydrates (white bread is out; wheat bread is in), while sugar is completely eliminated and organic whole foods are encouraged. Eating processed foods is discouraged.

How it Works

In addition to promoting the consumption of the right kind of fats, the Hamptons Diet also advises to avoid processed foods, which are the foods that promote chronic diseases like diabetes, cancer, obesity, and heart disease. Processed foods often contain trans-fatty acids, the ones now related to cancer more than saturated fats. Manufactured, brand-name foods are not considered healthy foods. The way to eat healthy is to purchase ingredients in bulk, like vegetables, fresh meats, and fruits, then prepare them yourself. Where possible, the food should be organic. With the right recipes, you don't need to be a chef to make healthy meals fast.

Advantages

- The Hamptons Diet, unlike other low-carbohydrate diets, does not promote the consumption of unhealthy fats like animal fat (saturated fat), hydrogenated oils, and soybean oil, which is high in omega-6 fatty acids.
- Macadamia oil is a superb nutritional source that reduces the risk of heart disease, cancer, and diabetes, and can help keep cholesterol levels at bay.
- The Hamptons Diet does promote weight loss.
- The elimination of processed foods is also a good thing.

Disadvantages

- Ingredients are so upscale you need to be able to afford to live in the Hamptons to afford this diet.

Summary

As far as popular low-carbohydrate diets go, the Hamptons Diet seems to have some sensible advice—particularly compared with the Atkins Diet. The diet encourages dieters to shift to a more balanced range of foods including monounsaturated fats, complex carbohydrates, and no processed foods, which is a step in the right direction. However, nutritionists believe it cuts way back on healthful foods like fruits, vegetables, and dairy. On the flip side, unlike other low-carbohydrate diets that encourage the widespread consumption of saturated fats, the Hamptons Diet places a lot of emphasis on consuming the right kind of fats—specifically monounsaturated fats.

23

Hay Diet

Overview

The Hay Diet created by Dr. William Hay, is known as a "food-combining diet" and is based on the premise of not mixing proteins with carbohydrates. This in turn aids digestion and facilitates weight loss, and keeps the digestive system healthy. This conclusion was drawn from the fact that the eating habits of our ancestors were not as complex as they are today, and since we evolved from them, changing our eating habits to those of our ancestors will reduce unwanted gains in body fat as seen in the age of the caveman.

How it Works

The Hay Diet consists of six basic rules:

1. Starches and sugars should not be eaten with proteins or acid fruits at the same meal.
2. Vegetables, salads, and fruits (whether acid or sweet), if correctly combined, should form the major part of the diet.
3. Proteins, starches, and fats should be eaten only in small quantities.
4. Eat only whole grains and unprocessed starches, and exclude refined, processed foods such as white flour, white sugar, and margarine.
5. Allow at least four hours between meals of different types.
6. Milk does not combine well with food and should be kept to a minimum.

Advantages

-   The Hay Diet can reverse chronic and degenerative conditions such as constipation, indigestion and arthritis.

- It can be beneficial to asthma and allergy sufferers.
- The Hay Diet can also stimulate natural weight loss, thus reducing the health risks linked to obesity, such as diabetes, gallstones, and coronary heart disease.
- The diet recommends eating more whole-grain foods, fruit, and vegetables, which is a good thing in any case.

Disadvantages

- The Hay Diet can be hard to follow as there are many complicated charts outlining the do's and don'ts.
- Lacking firm scientific basis, many food-combining diets provide inadequate vitamins and minerals. Protein and carbohydrates cannot be eaten together, so people have to choose one or the other. As a result, people often consume more carbohydrates than protein, as carbohydrates tend to be more filling and satisfying. Special care should be taken to ensure adequate intake of protein, calcium, zinc, vitamin D, and vitamin B12.
- Food-combining diets may fall below minimum recommended calorie levels.

Summary

The Hay Diet first gained credence as a method of weight loss since most dietary restrictions usually mean consuming fewer calories than the body needs. Hence it is no better than any other diet that is low in calories.

Scientifically, the Hay Diet is impossible to achieve since most starchy foods, such as bread and potatoes, contain some protein. The body is well adapted to digest both proteins and starch, and the enzymes necessary to digest them are secreted in response to the food being in the stomach.

The Hay Diet should always be avoided by anyone who has diabetes since carbohydrates should be spread evenly throughout the day and not kept to one meal only.

24

High-Fiber Diets

Overview

Most Americans consume far less fiber than their grandparents did, and as other countries modernize, the traditional fiber diets are discarded in favor of meat and more refined foods. Even the old sources of fiber are transformed by modern processing methods into foods that are virtually fiber-free. Although Americans still eat plenty of wheat, it is usually in the form of white bread, pizza, pastry, and some highly processed breakfast cereals whose fiber content is virtually nothing.

Dietary fiber—also known as roughage or bulk—is found in plant foods such as fruits, vegetables, whole grains and legumes that your body can't digest or absorb. Fiber is classified into two categories: those that don't dissolve in water (insoluble fiber), and those that do (soluble fiber).

Insoluble fiber moves through your digestive system more quickly than its counterpart. Insoluble fiber helps to keep the digestive system in good working order by increasing the bulk and softness of the stools, which in turn assists the smooth passage of food through the body. It's this type of fiber that helps to prevent bowel complaints like constipation and cancer. Foods rich in insoluble fiber include whole-wheat flour, nuts, vegetables, brown rice, bran, and fruits with edible seeds such as raspberries.

In contrast, soluble fiber is thought to bind with cholesterol and prevent it from being reabsorbed into the bloodstream. This lowers the amount of cholesterol in the blood, thereby reducing the risk of heart disease. Soluble fiber also forms a gel-like material in the intestine, which is thought to slow down the digestion and absorption of carbohydrates, especially glucose. This means it can help to keep blood sugar levels steady, preventing feelings of hunger. Foods rich in soluble fiber include oats, barley, apples, citrus fruits, carrots, and pulses such as beans, lentils, and peas.

How it Works

Good sources of fiber include whole-grain breads, rye bread, whole-wheat crackers, whole-grain or bran cereals, oatmeal (bran or grits), barley (dry), wheat germ, whole-wheat pasta, and brown rice. The best vegetable sources of fiber are the leafy vegetables: asparagus, celery, broccoli, Brussels sprouts, cabbage, cauliflower, and lettuce. Root vegetables like carrots, radishes, and turnips also have high amounts of fiber, as do yams, beans, peas, and corn. White potatoes contain fiber, although most of it is in their skins. Fiber-rich fruits include those with tough skins like apples and pears; those with fibrous interiors, like peaches; and those with edible seeds like blueberries and blackberries. Nuts are a particularly good source of fiber.

Refined or processed foods—such as fruit juice, white bread and pasta, and non-whole-grain cereals—are lower in fiber content. The refining process removes the outer layer of the kernel (bran) and the endosperm from grain, which lowers its fiber content. Similarly, removing the skin from fruits and vegetables decreases their fiber content.

Advantages

- High-Fiber diets have been shown to lower the risk of colon-rectal cancer, the second leading cause of cancer death in the U.S. and the second most common cancer for both sexes. Some medical experts theorize that the slower "transit time" of low-fiber diets may allow intestinal bacteria more time to multiply and keep them in longer contact with the intestinal walls; the prolonged exposure may produce cancer-causing substances or create an environment in which such substances flourish.

- Foods that contain fiber also tend to contain other cancer fighting nutrients, such as vitamin A, vitamin C, vitamin E, and selenium.

- Studies have shown that increased fiber helps ward off heart disease and heart attacks, and lowers cholesterol.

- This diet can be used in relieving symptoms, in the prevention or treatment of small pouches in your colon (diverticular disease), hemorrhoids, constipation, Crohn's disease, hypercholesterol-emia, obesity, and irritable bowel syndrome.

- It will soften up the food in your stomach as well as promote healthy stools.

- Researchers have demonstrated that high-fiber diets protect against gastroesophageal reflux disease (GERD). GERD, or acid reflux, leads to symptoms of acid indigestion, which affects about one in five Americans. Most people have GERD when the esophagus comes in contact with stomach acids. Left untreated, GERD can lead to ulcers and bleeding of the esophagus. It can also increase the risk of cancer of the esophagus.

- High-fiber diets may slow the absorption of sugar, which, for people with diabetes, may decrease the need for insulin. A high-fiber diet may also reduce the risk of developing Type 2 diabetes (formerly called adult-onset or noninsulin-dependent diabetes).

- Eating a high-fiber diet may also help with weight control. High-fiber foods generally require more chewing time, which gives your body time to register when you're no longer hungry, so you're less likely to overeat. Also, a high-fiber diet tends to make a meal feel larger and linger longer, so you stay full for a greater amount of time. And high-fiber diets tend to be less "energy dense," which means they have fewer calories for the same volume of food.

Disadvantages

- High-fiber diets are good for your health, but too much fiber eaten too quickly can cause intestinal gas, abdominal bloating, and cramping. To minimize this, increase fiber in your diet gradually over a period of a few weeks. This allows the natural bacteria in your digestive system to adjust to the change. Also, drink plenty of water. Fiber works best when it absorbs water, making your stool soft and bulky. Without the added water, you could become constipated.

- Plant fiber may tie up calcium, magnesium, and zinc, preventing their absorption by the body. This should not be a problem for well-nourished individuals. However, athletes who undergo strenuous exercising may lose large quantities of zinc in sweat. If they are also on a high-fiber diet, they run the risk of zinc depletion and should increase their intake of foods rich in zinc.

Summary

Most nutritionists are big fans of high-fiber diets, not just because they can help to reduce the risk of health problems ranging from constipation to heart disease and cancer, but also because they may also help with weight control.

25

High Protein Diets

Overview

High protein diets, otherwise known as low-carbohydrates diets, are based on the concept that it may be healthier to eat more high protein foods such as meat, fish, and eggs, and limit high-carbohydrate foods. These diets have a high level of appeal to many people. The inventors of these diets make different claims about their effects on health, ranging from weight loss to massive reduction in disease risk and vastly increased life expectancy. Some of the more common high protein-low carbohydrate diets are:

The Atkins Diet

Hamptons Diet

Stillman Diet

Scarsdale Diet

Hollywood Diet

Ketogenic Diet

Zone Diet

The theory behind high protein diets is that slower-burning energy sources—protein and fat—provide a steady supply of energy and thus are less likely to lead to weight gain. In addition, people tend to feel full longer after eating protein than after eating carbohydrates, because carbohydrates empty from the stomach quickly and are digested quickly. Carbohydrates also strongly stimulate insulin production, which promotes fat deposition and increases appetite.

High protein diets can cause a quick drop in weight because eliminating carbohydrates causes a loss of body fluids. The increase in the amount of protein consumed, such as from meat and dairy products, forces the body into "starvation mode," which happens because the brain typically prefers to run on glucose (blood sugar) that is supplied by digested carbohydrate.

When there are not enough carbohydrates to convert into blood sugar, the body is forced to use some of its glycogen stored in the liver and muscles to maintain a normal blood sugar level. This process results in initial protein tissue (muscle) loss and urinary loss of electrolytes. Because muscle is mostly water, one will lose weight very rapidly in the first few days. If the carbohydrate restriction is prolonged, the brain eventually will run on fat stores for fuel (called ketosis). The amount of weight loss depends on the amount of fat one has stored.

How it Works

There are various versions of high protein diets. However, most recommend large quantities of protein in unrestricted amounts, including red meat, fish, shellfish, poultry, eggs, and cheese. Some of these diets recommend avoiding foods with a high glycemic index. Foods that contain carbohydrates are given a glycemic index, which indicates how quickly the carbohydrates are digested and thus how a food affects the level of sugar in the blood. Foods that contain large amounts of sugar (such as maple syrup, honey, and candy) and starchy foods (such as carrots, potatoes, and some cereals) have a high glycemic index because they are quickly digested and quickly increase blood sugar levels. Foods that are high in fiber (such as whole-grain rye bread and all-bran cereals) have a low glycemic index because they are digested more slowly and do not quickly increase blood sugar levels.

Advantages

- High protein diets lead to faster-than-average initial weight loss.
- Eating a high-protein diet may lead to a steadying of blood sugar levels.

Disadvantages

- Some high protein diets de-emphasize high-carbohydrate, high-fiber plant foods. These foods help lower cholesterol when eaten as part of a nutritionally balanced diet. Reducing consumption of these foods usually means other, higher-fat foods are eaten instead, which raises cholesterol levels even more and increases cardiovascular risk.

- Most Americans already eat more protein than their bodies need and eating too much protein can increase health risks. High-protein animal foods are usually also high in saturated fat and eating large amounts of high-fat foods for a sustained period raises the risk of coronary heart disease, diabetes, stroke and several types of cancer.

- People who can't use excess protein effectively may be at higher risk of kidney and liver disorders, and osteoporosis.

- High-protein diets don't provide some essential vitamins, minerals, fiber and other nutritional elements.

- A high-carbohydrate diet that includes fruits, vegetables, nonfat dairy products, and whole grains also has been shown to reduce blood pressure. Thus, limiting these foods may raise blood pressure by reducing the intake of calcium, potassium, and magnesium while simultaneously increasing sodium intake.

- High protein diets may encourage over-consumption of saturated fat and cholesterol, which can increase the risk of heart disease.

- There are numerous metabolic and health risks associated with ketosis, including fatigue in late afternoon, hypotension (too-low blood pressure), headaches, constipation, diarrhea, thinning hair, dry skin, altered breath, and muscle cramps.

Summary

Most of these high protein diets aren't balanced in terms of the essential nutrients our bodies need. Some of these diets emphasize foods like meat, eggs, and cheese, which are rich in protein and saturated fat. While others restrict healthful foods that provide essential nutrients and don't provide the variety of foods needed to adequately meet nutritional needs. Some restrict important carbohydrates such as cereals, grains, fruits, vegetables, and low-fat dairy products. People who stay on these diets very long may not get enough vitamins and minerals, and face other potential health risks. Some evidence suggests that over years, very high protein diets impair kidney function and may contribute to the decrease in kidney function that occurs in older people. People with certain kidney and liver disorders should not consume a high-protein diet.

Dieticians do not consider the glycemic index a useful tool for dieters. The difference between the speed of carbohydrate digestion for foods with the highest and lowest glycemic indexes is so small that it makes little difference to most dieters. Avoiding foods with a high glycemic index does not promote weight loss, and as mentioned it eliminates foods with valuable vitamins and minerals.

Although everyone agrees high protein-low carbohydrate diets cause weight loss during the first week or so, as the body converts stored carbohydrates (glycogen) to energy. Nutritionists contend that once the body begins to use stored fat for energy, weight loss slows.

26

Jenny Craig Diet

Overview

In 1983, Jenny Craig started her first commercial weight loss program in Australia by providing frozen and shelf-stable prepared meals to help with portion management and calorie-intake control. Today Jenny Craig has 800 centers, making it one of the largest weight management programs in the world. If you don't have a Jenny Craig Weight Loss Centre near you, or if you prefer to go it alone you can try Jenny Direct, her at-home program. Developed by certified professionals in medicine, registered dietitians, and psychologists, the program focuses on a lifestyle and holistic approach, such as incorporating exercise into your daily life and building a healthy relationship with food. Jenny Craig has also branched out into cookbooks and programs that encourage clients to make food choices from readily available foods.

The Jenny Craig Diet program relies on your purchase of a variety of pre-packaged foods, eventually progressing to preparing your own foods with healthy menus. The food selections look enticing, offering meals such as Island Style Chicken, Traditional Lasagna, and even Double Chocolate Cake for dessert. The nutritional content of the meals is comparable to *Healthy Choice* or *Lean Cuisine* frozen meals that are available in every supermarket at reasonable prices. In addition to membership fees and food costs for Jenny Craig prepackaged meals, you are responsible for additional food choices, such as perishable items.

With individual counseling and prepackaged meals, the program leaves little to chance or to the dieter's discretion. The program helps dieters set realistic weight-loss goals and then helps in crafting a plan to successfully achieve that goal. The Jenny Craig program says it teaches you how to man-age food, feelings, and fitness. Jenny Craig believes that the combination of complete support, step-by-step instruction about what to eat, and con-trolled portions during the initial dieting stage together help dieters win at weight loss.

How it Works

The Jenny Craig Diet program is a three-phase plan to help people lose weight and keep it off. The first phase of the program teaches clients how to eat the foods they want—in small, frequent portions. The second phase of the program teaches clients how to increase their energy levels via simple activity. The third phase of the program teaches clients how to build more balance into their lives in order to maintain weight loss and a healthy diet.

Jenny Craig requires that you initially purchase and eat Jenny Craig prepared entrees and snacks at every meal. Nutritionally, they're based on the USDA food pyramid and contain 60% carbohydrate, 20% protein, and 20% fat. There is a wide variety of dishes to choose from, including sweet and sour chicken, beef sirloin dinner, chicken fettuccine, pancakes, vegetarian sausage, raspberry swirl cheesecake, and double chocolate cake. Dieters can supplement these meals with fresh fruits and vegetables, whole grains, and low-fat dairy products. Eventually, after losing enough weight, you can begin the transition to supermarket food, using a food diary to record everything you eat.

All foods are allowed, but the focus of the Jenny Craig Diet is on moderation, a balanced diet, and getting enough exercise. But built into the program are occasional splurges that allow dieters to indulge themselves a little.

That being said, the Jenny Craig Diet program is calorie based. The menus a client develops with his or her counselor are based on an individual's weight, height, and goals. The number of calories consumed every day is calculated according to your height and weight, but you are not allowed to go below a minimum of 1,000 calories. Diet plans are also available for vegetarians, people with diabetes, and those who observe kosher dietary laws.

The program offers several levels of support, such as its 24/7 telephone line, allowing clients to get information and support when they need it. The program also offers online support, including peer-support discussion groups. A wide variety of written materials are also available for support.

Advantages

- The Jenny Craig Diet program offers counseling on food issues and nutrition.

- Using frozen meals is convenient, and the meals are balanced and nutritious.

- There are many options to make the menu planning flexible and individualized.

- The individual weekly behavior consultations promote lifestyle changes and give on going support.

- The Jenny Craig Diet program is good for losing weight.

Disadvantages

- The Jenny Craig Diet is low in fiber, possibly due to limited choices of whole-grain foods. Some daily menu plans may also be low in iron, zinc and vitamin E.

- The Jenny Craig Diet relies on a food exchange system for menu planning, which many people find cumbersome and confusing.

- Most people find that eating prepackaged foods tends to be boring.

- Dieters on the Jenny Craig Diet are required to buy their food from Jenny Craig. This is convenient, but can get a bit pricey.

- The Jenny Craig Diet program requires packaged meals, which is not conducive for teaching clients how to shop, cook, and eat their own healthy, calorie-controlled meals. Hence, dieters who resume their usual eating habit are likely to regain weight after completing the Jenny Craig Diet program.

- Some clients may have difficulty eating Jenny Craig packaged meals long-term, especially during periods of travel, social dining, or illness.

- Jenny Craig counselors have no formal training in weight loss management.

- Group meetings are not offered at Jenny Craig franchises, but on-line "chat" groups are available to clients.

Summary

If you want to lose some weight fairly quickly, the Jenny Craig Diet can get you on the right path in a short period of time. The prescribed diet is easy to follow, balanced, and nutritious; however, the diet can be quite expensive, especially for those with a low budget.

Prices vary depending on your individual choices, but the company says the average cost is about $65 a week, including entrees and snacks. Jenny Craig offers three membership options: platinum, gold, and special promotional memberships, which are frequently offered. Depending on the type of membership and which meals and snacks eaten, it can cost about $400 during the first month of the program. Jenny Craig does offer and encourage members to purchase its own brand of vitamin and mineral supplements; however, they are not required as part of the diet program. The program also sells audio cassettes for walkers and a fitness video series to help you incorporate physical activity into your daily routine.

The Jenny Craig Diet is good for teaching portion control, but many nutritionists question the value of learning portion control from prepackaged foods. They believe once you go off the packaged meals it is difficult to translate those portions of food back to a semblance of normal eating.

Nutritionists point out that, while the counselors are trained to be Jenny Craig counselors, they are not nutritionists.

27

Jorge Cruise Diet

Overview

Jorge Cruise is the author of *8 Minutes in the Morning*, which was written to help you jump start your metabolism and begin burning more calories. The diet program involves an eight-minute weight-bearing exercise every day designed to strengthen and work particular muscle groups. Add to this a really easy-to-follow diet plan focused around portion control, and emphasizing eating vegetables and fruits, whole grains and fewer white refined carbohydrates, and you have a very easy plan for improving health, losing excess body fat, and feeling better than you have in years.

Cruise guarantees that by following the simple exercise and diet plan you can lose two pounds a week.

How it Works

The 28-day diet program involves just two different strength-training exercises every morning for only eight minutes (four minutes for each exercise). The pair of exercises always works two major muscle groups. For example, Monday is devoted to chest and back, while Tuesday concentrates on the shoulders and abdominals.

The routines focus on strength training, which Cruise says is the number-one exercise when it comes to weight loss. Strength training builds lean muscle tissue, which boosts your metabolism, burning more calories not only when exercising but throughout the day. The single most important factor that determines how much fat you burn throughout the day is the amount of lean muscle tissue in your body.

Another component of Cruise's plan is a diet that controls portions and emphasizes filling foods, such as healthful fats, complex carbohydrates, and vegetables, plus lots of water. The program is very similar to the South Beach Diet, but this plan gives you a set number of calories per day—between

1,200 and 2,000 calories—depending on our weight. To make it easy, the book includes an Eating Card System, which is to be copied for daily use. The cards include check boxes for each necessary food component to help track daily intake.

The third, and perhaps most important, key is recognizing what Cruise describes as "self-sabotage"—eating for emotional reasons instead of true hunger. Cruise outlines three steps for eliminating emotional eating:

1. Identify the emotion.
2. Identify the opposite emotion.
3. Create a new plan to invoke this opposite emotion more in your life.

Advantages

- The Jorge Cruise Diet guarantees that by following the simple exercise and diet plan you can lose two pounds a week.
- The diet promotes daily exercise.
- There's a welcome emphasis on whole grains, fruits and vegetables that is lacking in many diet plans.
- The diet encourages eating all the types of foods known to prevent heart disease, including nuts, monounsaturated fats like olive and canola oil, soy products, whole grains, and fruits and vegetables.

Disadvantages

- Cruise's nutritional advice is often misleading.

Summary

Nutritionists for the most part believe the diet plan offers some good diet strategies—exercising and eating a healthy balance diet. However, they think the program misleads dieters when it says that eight minutes of exercise builds enough muscle to burn fat. The amount of exercise is considered small, and it's probably the smaller portions or low calorie foods that are making dieters lose weight—not the exercise. They also question some of Cruise's nutrition advice, such as his opinions about flaxseed oil and his comments about dairy foods causing sinus problems.

28

Kashi GOLEAN Diet

Overview

Kashi offers a wide range of foods (shakes, cereals, crackers and snack bars) to enable people to achieve optimal health, wellness, and weight management goals. When it comes to weight loss and management, Kashi's GOLEAN line of high fiber and low fat products offers cereals that are rich in protein, fiber, and soy, as well as shakes and snack bars, in a variety of flavors and sizes. All Kashi foods are natural, minimally processed, and free of highly refined sugars, artificial additives, and preservatives.

How it Works

A typical plan includes eating Kashi GOLEAN foods throughout the day for breakfast, lunch, and an afternoon snack followed by a healthy and nutritious meal of your choice for dinner.

Advantages

- Kashi GOLEAN foods are low in fat and high in fiber.
- They make great use of whole grains and soy protein for added nutritional benefits to help you eat healthy while losing weight.
- The company also provides lots of useful nutrition and weight loss information in their brochures and on their website.

Disadvantages

- Relying solely on Kashi GOLEAN products can get old quickly, even with their variety of flavors.
- The high-fiber diet may cause gas or bloating.
- The Kashi GOLEAN diet requires continuous purchase of their products for the duration of your diet.

Summary

Overall, the Kashi GOLEAN Diet is a nutritionally balanced weight-loss plan. Typically people who follow the program over a period of time will loss weight. On average, participants lost only small amounts of weight while on the diet, but some participants have been known to lose considerably more weight, with the maximum amount of weight loss reaching around 50 pounds.

Life Choice Diet

Overview

The Life Choice Diet by Dr. Dean Ornish is a low-fat, vegetarian diet that focuses on lowering blood cholesterol levels, body weight, incidence of cancer, heart disease, arthritis, and other diseases. The diet emphasizes the consumption of whole grains, beans, fruits and vegetables, and severely restricts the consumption of animal products, dietary fat, and refined carbohydrates.

All foods containing cholesterol and saturated fats are prohibited from the diet. Saturated fats are found in meat, dairy products, oils, nuts, seeds, and avocados, which are all forbidden by the Life Choice Diet. The level of polyunsaturated fat in the diet is reduced to only 10% of the total calories. This level is much lower for diets recommended by the American Heart Association, which recommends about 30% of calories from fat. The typical American diet can contain as much as 50% fat.

How it Works

The Life Choice Diet is 10% fat, 20% protein, and 70% carbohydrates. The Life Choice Diet encourages eating complex carbohydrates such as whole grains, vegetables, fruits, legumes, and soybean products in unlimited quantities. The diet restricts, but does not eliminate, simple carbohydrates such as sugar and honey. Individuals following the diet must avoid all meat and dairy products, except egg whites, nonfat milk, and nonfat yogurt. Egg whites are a source of protein on the diet. To adhere to the strict limitation on dietary fat intake, individuals on the Life Choice Diet must restrict their consumption of plant foods that contain high amounts of fat, including all vegetable oils, nuts, seeds, and avocados.

The Life Choice Diet recommends a spectrum of foods grouped from beneficial to least beneficial, based mainly on fat and cholesterol content. Group 1 foods, those that are most beneficial, include whole grains, beans, fruits, and vegetables. Group 2 foods, foods that should be eaten only in moderation, include nonfat diary products such as skim milk, nonfat yogurt, and egg whites, plus other nonfat or very low-fat commercially available products. Foods that should be eaten sparingly fall into Group 3, and include foods like oils, low-fat diary products, fish, maple syrup, and honey. Group 4 foods, such poultry, all shellfish, and refined sugar products should be avoided when possible. Group 5 foods should be avoided altogether, and range from beef and pork products to fried chicken, coconut oil, egg yolks, whole milk foods, salt, caffeinated beverages, and alcohol.

Dieters are encouraged to graze throughout the day rather than eating three big meals.

In addition to these dietary recommendations, the Life Choice Diet involves comprehensive lifestyle changes including moderate aerobic exercise, stress reduction techniques (such as stretching, meditation, and imagery), peer support, smoking cessation, and nutritional supplementation (with folic acid, vitamin C, vitamin E, vitamin B12, fish oil, flaxseed oil, and selenium).

Advantages

- The Life Choice Diet has also been shown to be an effective weight loss program.
- Dieters won't feel deprived on the Life Choice Diet because they can eat generous amounts of fresh plant foods that are naturally low in fat without having to count calories.
- Ornish suggests that his diet plan can help dieters increase their metabolism.
- The Life Choice Diet is recommended as a preventive measure for heart disease, strokes, diabetes, and other conditions related to high fat consumption.

Disadvantages

- The Life Choice Diet has a very restricted menu, making the diet too pristine for a majority of people.

- The diet plan is deficient in vitamin E, vitamin B12, vitamin D, and calcium due to its low fat content and its de-emphasis on meat and few dairy foods, respectively.

- High volume of fiber-rich foods (fiber content of the Life Choice Diet is nearly twice that recommended by the USDA Food Guide Pyramid) may cause gastrointestinal distress and decreased nutrient absorption in the gut.

- Avoidance of sugar, salt, and fat, primary flavoring agents in the American diet, may be unpalatable for some dieters.

- Fat also gives us a feeling of satiety, meaning it helps us feel satisfied, curbs our appetite, and guards against overeating. People who follow a very-low-fat diet often feel hungry and unsatisfied.

- Daily consumption of fresh, unprocessed foods promoted by the Life Choice Diet can be an ongoing challenge for dieters who have little time to cook, travel often for business or dine out socially.

Summary

A vegetarian diet is best for overall health with vegetarians as a group having lower cholesterol, weigh less, and suffer less chronic disease than their meat-eating counterparts. However, some nutritionists wonder whether the diet is too low in fat, and believe the diet does not provide a sufficient amount of essential fatty acids, all of which are critical to good health. The Life Choice Diet excludes fish, despite a significant body of research that demonstrates a protective effect of fish (and fish oil) consumption against heart disease. And the diet's high carbohydrate levels may pose a problem for people with diabetes or those who are resistant to insulin—albeit this is a small part of the population.

30

Liver Cleansing Diet

Overview

The Liver Cleansing Diet, developed by Dr. Sandra Cabot, is based on the premise that the liver is the gateway to maintaining a healthy body. Cabot lists the many symptoms of Liver Dysfunction, which range from bad breath to allergies, from menstrual problems to obesity, and from autoimmune diseases to chronic fatigue.

By following her diet, while also taking nutritional supplements and "liver tonics" you will (she claims) experience increased energy levels, detoxification and cleansing of the blood stream, reduction of inflammation and degenerative diseases, better immune function, more efficient fat metabolism, and weight control.

How it Works

The Liver Cleansing Diet is an eight-week eating plan to detoxify and reduce fat levels in the liver. The diet consists of a series of recipes that Cabot provides (available only in her books). The diet plan cuts out sugar and most processed food products. Red meat and dairy are also removed from the diet. The diet concentrates on eating lots of raw fruit, vegetables, and juices. Legumes, grains, seeds, and nuts are combined as protein sources and snacks. Organic chicken and eggs are allowed (though not in the middle four weeks).

Taking Livatone powder or capsules will increase the ability of the liver to detoxify itself.

While there are numerous recipes to follow, simply combining allowable protein foods with salads, vegetables, pastas, or rice for lunches and dinners is quick and easy. Juices, smoothies, muesli, fruit, toast, and spreads are breakfast options.

Advantages

- The Liver Cleansing Diet increases energy levels.
- It detoxifies and cleanses the blood stream.
- It results in a reduction of inflammation and degenerative diseases.
- The diet improves the body's immune function.
- It results in efficient fat metabolism.
- The diet has been known to result in weight loss.

Disadvantages

- The Liver Cleansing Diet is so restrictive (eating only raw fruits and vegetables), it will not appeal to many people.
- There is no proof that supplements and "liver tonics" will work.

Summary

The scientific evidence that particular foods will specifically target the liver and 'cleanse' it is virtually non-existent. It is certainly true that the liver is involved in many processes that impact on health, including detoxifying poisons such as alcohol, but to describe the liver as 'the gateway to the body' is perhaps an exaggeration. Proper functioning of all organs—including the brain, heart, pancreas, stomach and kidneys, among others—and not just the liver, is essential for health and well-being.

Despite this, Cabot manages to give mostly appropriate dietary advice, even though it may be inappropriately directed specifically at improving liver function. Consistent with current nutritional concepts, her diet is largely based on high intakes of fruits and vegetables (although she inappropriately recommends eating only the raw forms of these); a wide range of protein sources, including lean meat, fish, legumes, grains, nuts, and seeds; minimizing saturated fat consumption; and moderating consumption of sugars.

Unfortunately, the advice also includes taking many nutritional supplements and liver tonics. There is little or no scientific evidence supporting the value of this advice. Some supplements are considered to be potentially dangerous, and in any case, supplements are unlikely to be beneficial if your diet is based on a wide range of nutritious foods. Finally, there is little or no scientific evidence that liver tonics will have beneficial effects specifically on the liver (or on any other organ).

Cabot also neglects to stress the importance of physical activity in promoting and maintaining health and wellness.

Although the Liver Cleansing Diet contains some valuable dietary advice, it is not based on sound science and cannot be recommended for either the short or long term.

31

Living Low-Carb Diet

Overview

The Living Low-Carb Diet is the brainchild of Fran McCullough, an author and award-winning cookbook editor. Struggling to keep her own weight down, McCullough was led to a low-carbohydrate diet, which she put together in a collection of more than 250 recipes in the *The Low-Carb Cookbook*. She later came out with the *Living Low-Carb* book, which contains more explanations about dieting and adds another 175 recipes. Rather than just a "diet" book, *Living Low-Carb* is more of a lifestyle and self-help guide with recipes for everything from home fries to Moroccan-styled chicken to what she calls Intense Chocolate Cake.

McCullough dismisses the raft of objections levied at her low-carbohydrate diet by the nutritional establishment, but she does note that for some people this type of routine is not ideal. She discusses the particular needs of diabetics and those with low-thyroid function, and includes caveats for those pregnant or nursing. The Living Low-Carb Diet is full of motivational suggestions, as well as practical advice for stocking the pantry; eating on the road, in restaurants, and at the homes of friends; and finally, how to deal with a dieter's bete noir, the sweet tooth.

The diet encourages exercise—not because it will make you lose fat, but because it's good for you—and gives you more than a dozen reasons why you should exercise.

How it Works

Instead of a concrete diet plan, the Living Low-Carb Diet is more of a tool to help you weigh the pros and cons of eating low-carbohydrates. If you're looking for precise food lists and specific menus, you're out of luck. But if you're pondering the feasibility of eating low-carbohydrates, you may find some valuable tips.

The plan recommends drinking 8 to 12 cups of water daily. Eat protein at every meal—about one-half gram of protein for every pound of your ideal weight, typically somewhere between 60 and 85 grams unless you're very large or very small. If you want to lose weight eat fewer carbohydrates, anywhere from zero to 30 grams daily. Preferably it is better to eat whole-grian foods—organic if possible, and raw, ideally. Avoid foods such as potatoes, rice, bread, flour, sugar, or popcorn. Eat fruit at breakfast, particularly low-carbohydrate fruits such as berries, melons, peaches, and kiwi. Although you are allowed cream and butter, save it for treats, and cut down on them if you are trying to lose weight. Choose cold-pressed olive and nut oils, and avoid processed oils, partially hydrogenated fats, and margarine. Eat dinner early and make it minimal.

Advantages

- The primary benefit of the Living Low-Carb Diet is rapid and substantial weight loss.

- Some research indicates that people with Type 2 diabetes have better insulin function and better blood sugar control on a low carbohydrate diet.

- Because you can eat as much as you like of the permitted foods, there is reduced fatigue.

- Considered to lower risk for chronic illnesses, like heart disease, high blood pressure, and diabetes.

Disadvantages

- The Living Low-Carb Diet also promotes L-carnitine and liver-cleansing supplements, neither of which are proven weight-loss aids.

- There is concern with the diet's "emergency fast pound drop" regimen, which tells dieters to cut or drastically limit whole food groups (such as fruits and dairy) that provide key nutrients.

Summary

Nutritionists are wary of promoting low-carbohydrate, high-protein diets since there is a lack in food choices and the resulting difficulty that some people have staying within the limited choices over the long term. Also, there is concern over the lack of data on the long-term safety and effectiveness of low-carbohydrate diets, especially by those who may have a preclinical or "silent" condition or illness. To lose weight, medical experts recommend a diet low in saturated fat, and high in fruits, vegetables, and high-fiber-containing carbohydrates.

32

Macrobiotic Diet

Overview

The word "macrobiotic" comes from Greek roots and means "long life." The Macrobiotic Diet was developed by a Japanese educator named George Ohsawa, who believed that simplicity was the key to optimal health. Michio Kushi expanded on Ohsawa's macrobiotic theory and opened the Kushi Institute in Boston in 1978. Together with his wife, Aveline, Kushi published many books on macrobiotics and was responsible for popularizing the diet in North America.

At the core of macrobiotics is the concept of yin and yang—forces which Oriental philosophers believe must be kept in harmony to achieve good health. In Chinese philosophy, the opposing forces of yin and yang govern all aspects of life. Yin—representative of an outward centrifugal movement—results in expansion. On the other hand, yang—representative of an inward centripetal movement—produces contraction. In addition, yin is said to be cold while yang is hot; yin is sweet, yang is salty; yin is passive and yang is aggressive. In the macrobiotic view, the forces of yin and yang must be kept in balance to achieve good health.

To the extent that these qualities are reflected in food, the macrobiotic dietary regimen strives to achieve harmony between yin and yang. Certain foods are said to be very yin, others very yang, and some are in between. For example, foods considered to be very yin include sugar, tea, alcohol, coffee, milk, cream, yogurt, and most herbs and spices. Foods that are considered to be very yang include red meat, poultry, fish and shellfish, eggs, hard cheeses, and salt. Foods that are thought to contain a harmonious balance in the yin/yang continuum (though not necessarily in nutritional science) are brown rice and whole grains. Hence, those foods constitute the foundation of the macrobiotic diet. Eating those foods is thought to make it easier to achieve a more balanced condition within the natural order of life. Foods that are considered either extremely yin or extremely yang are to be avoided.

The Macrobiotic Diet is appealing to health-minded individuals who are seeking a holistic approach to physical and spiritual well-being. The Macrobiotic Diet is a low-fat, high fiber diet that is a predominantly vegetarian diet, emphasizing whole grains and vegetables. In addition, the Macrobiotic Diet is rich in phytoestrogens from soy products.

How it Works

The macrobiotic regimen adds foods reflecting different degrees of yin and yang, selected in accordance with the individual's dietary needs and temperament. In practice, this usually works out to a diet consisting of the following food categories.

Whole Grains

Whole grains including brown rice, barley, millet, oats, corn, rye, whole wheat, and buckwheat are believed to be the most balanced foods on the yin/yang continuum, and should comprise 50–60% of a person's daily food intake. Although whole grains are preferred, breads must at least be made without yeast. Pasta is allowed in small amounts.

Vegetables

Fresh vegetables should comprise 25–30% of food intake. Daily consumption of any of the following vegetables is highly recommended: cabbage, broccoli, cauliflower, kale, bok choi, collards, mustard greens, kohlrabi, turnips, turnip greens, rutabaga, onion, radishes, acorn squash, butternut squash, and pumpkin. Vegetables to be eaten occasionally (two to three times per week) include cucumbers, celery, iceberg lettuce, mushrooms, snow peas, and string beans. Potatoes, tomatoes, and eggplants are not permitted as they originated in tropical regions; when they are eaten in temperate climates it is believed to contribute to the loss of natural immunity.

Beans and sea vegetables should comprise 5–10% of daily food intake. Especially recommended are adzuki beans, chickpeas (garbanzo beans), lentils, and tofu. In this category, tofu (soybean curd) is a favorite. Sea vegetables, including wakame, hiziki, dombu, noris, arame, agar-agar, and Irish moss, are rich in many vitamins and minerals, and are easily added at each meal.

Soups

Soups and broths comprise 5–10% of food intake. Soups containing miso (soy bean paste), vegetables, and beans are acceptable.

Seeds, Nuts, and Fish

Seeds, nuts, and fish also comprise 5–10% of the diet. A few servings each week of seeds and nuts, sesame, sunflower and pumpkin seeds, peanuts, almonds, hazelnuts, walnuts, and dried chestnuts are permissible. For non-vegetarians, three small portions of fresh seafood (halibut, flounder, cod, or sole) can be included every week. The yang qualities of fish and shellfish should be balanced by eating green leafy vegetables, grains or pulses in the same meal.

Fruit

Fruit comprise about 5% of the diet. A mixture should contain fresh seasonal fruits, which should include some citrus fruit. Itis important to ensure freshness. If possible, choose local produce. The diet advises against eating fruits that are not grown locally such as bananas, pineapples, and other tropical fruits if you live in a temperate climate.

Condiments and Seasonings

Commonly used seasonings include natural sea salt, shoyu, brown rice vinegar, umeboshi vinegar, umeboshi plums, grated ginger root, garlic, fermented pickles, gomashio (roasted sesame seeds), roasted seaweed, sliced scallions, and tamari soy sauce. Brown rice syrup, barley malt, and amasake (a sweet rice drink) may be used as sweeteners.

Beverages

The beverages one should drink on the macrobiotic plan include spring or well water and any traditional tea that is without fragrance or stimulants. Only teas made from roasted grains, dandelion greens, or the cooking water of soba noodles are generally considered acceptable. Drinking and cooking water must be purified.

Restricted Foods

To maintain proper yin/yang balance, all extremely yang foods and all extremely yin foods should be avoided. All animal foods, including eggs and dairy products, are believed to have a strong yang quality. Extremely yin foods include some beverages, refined sugars, chocolate, tropical fruits, soda, fruit juice, colored and aromatic teas, coffee, strong alcohol, and hot spices. In addition, all foods processed with artificial colors, flavors, or preservatives must be avoided.

Food Preparation

Macrobiotic principles also govern food preparation and the manner in which food is eaten. Vegetables should be lightly steamed, boiled, or sautéed in vegetable oil and rice must be pressure-cooked. Since the objective is to get one to live in harmony with nature, electrical or microwave cooking is not recommended. Recommended cooking fuels are wood and natural gas. Wood utensils are allowed, while plastic utensils are to be avoided.

Advantages

- The Macrobiotic Diet is high in natural unrefined foods.
- Proponents assert that the balance and harmony of the Macrobiotic Diet and lifestyle create the best possible conditions for health. They claim that the diet yields many positive health effects, including a general sense of well-being.
- The Macrobiotic Diet encompasses many of the dietary elements linked to a reduced risk of pancreatic cancer and heart disease.

The diet is low in saturated fats, high in fiber, and rich in crucifer-ous vegetables and soy products.

- The macrobiotic emphasis on fresh, non-processed foods may help reduce or eliminate certain food allergies and chemical sensitivities.

- It would be difficult to gain weight or become obese by following a Macrobiotic Diet program.

Disadvantages

- Many nutrition experts disapprove of the limited number of foods allowed on the Macrobiotic Diet, but concede that a moderate approach to macrobiotics poses no real harm. However, strict macrobiotic diets can be deficient in calories, vitamin B12, vitamin D, calcium, and iron. As a result, this type of diet is not suitable for children or for pregnant or lactating women without appropriate supplementation.

- Food preparation techniques are rigidly prescribed and quite complicated and tedious.

- Many of the special foods recommended are not available locally, which is a weakness in suggesting that macrobiotic practitioners everywhere eat a similar diet.

- Perhaps most dangerous are the implications that the diet alone will cure the disease and that patients can and should avoid conventional medical therapy.

- A drawback to macrobiotics, especially for Americans, is that it requires an acceptance of Eastern philosophy—near religion, if you will—but at least a way of life that goes along with the diet.

Summary

Despite the purported benefits, few mainstream nutritionists endorse a strict Macrobiotic Diet. The Macrobiotic Diet discourages the intake of meat, fowl, and most fish—all of which provide protein and fat that is essential for development. The restrictive nature of macrobiotics designates food as good or bad. However, nutritionists maintain a balanced diet is essential in order to promote physiologic health. A wider variety of foods will provide a wider variety of vitamins and nutrients. A diet that excludes many foods eliminates the consumption of a variety of vitamins and minerals that are essential to a balanced diet. The selection of foods is so limited (often little more than brown rice and grain), nutritionists warn that you can easily develop significant nutritional deficiencies: protein, vitamin B12, vitamin D, calcium, and riboflavin.

Nutritionists also add that, while a Macrobiotic Diet may indeed reduce your risk of heart disease and cancer, it will not cure any specific disorder—including cancer. The American Cancer Society is aware of no diet that can cure cancer. Until more conclusive research is available on the health benefits of the Macrobiotic Diet, individuals with serious medical conditions such as cancer should continue to seek the support of qualified medical providers in conjunction with any dietary changes.

33

Mayo Clinic Diet

Overview

The Mayo Clinic Diet is not endorsed by the Mayo Clinic health centre and hospital in Rochester, Minnesota. The Mayo Clinic Diet was conceived 30 years ago, and its origins still remain unknown. Today it appears in many forms but one main characteristic of a Mayo Clinic Diet is that it usually contains grapefruit as a way to encourage your body to burn fat and is usually high in protein and low in carbohydrates.

The theory behind the Mayo Clinic Diet is that a low carbohydrate diet plan will result in quick weight loss.

How it Works

The Mayo Clinic Diet usually lasts anywhere between three and seven days, and generally does not exceed seven days in duration. While on the Mayo Clinic Diet, participants are allowed to eat an unlimited amount of grapefruit, meat, and poultry. All of the fat in this diet should counter your appetite so you shouldn't be very hungry for carbohydrate-loaded snacks. Complex carbohydrates are, for the most part, banned, and any other carbohydrate intake should be strictly limited.

Advantages

- The Mayo Clinic Diet may promote rapid weight loss.
- You get to eat as much meat as you want, and fried foods are actually encouraged.

Disadvantages

- This Mayo Clinic Diet simply does not work for long-term weight management.

- It contains no complex carbohydrates, and can cause physical weakness and lack of concentration.

- In the real world, the fat that we eat does not cause us to lose weight, and there is nothing in grapefruit that leads our body to begin using fat for energy.

- Unlimited consumption of anything high in fat can lead to increased risk of heart disease in the long-term.

Summary

Like many other diets, the Mayo Clinic Diet promotes temporary quick weight loss but is not necessarily safe or nutritionally balanced. Critics argue that the Mayo Clinic Diet does not contribute to long-term weight management. Health experts are skeptical of the Mayo Clinic Diet's claim of rapid weight loss and argue that grapefruit does not contain any fat-burning qualities. Although some dieticians do acknowledge that the Mayo Clinic Diet can result in rapid weight loss, it is usually only temporary. They also warn that the diet is not safe and should not be followed for any length of time.

34

Mediterranean Diet

Overview

The Mediterranean Diet is not a specific diet plan, rather it's a nutritional concept based on the dietary eating patterns of countries bordering the Mediterranean Sea. These cultures have eating habits that developed over thousands of years. People in Europe, parts of Italy, Greece, Portugal, Spain, and southern France adhere to principles of the Mediterranean Diet, as do people in Morocco and Tunisia in North Africa. Parts of the Balkan region and Turkey follow the diet, as well as Middle Eastern countries like Lebanon and Syria. Although there are many variations of the Mediterranean Diet, due to social, political, and economic differences between these countries they all share one common characteristic in their diet. They have diets that are low in saturated fat and high in omega-3 fatty acids and monounsaturated fats. The omega-3 fatty acids are found in fatty fish (e.g., salmon, trout, sardines, and tuna) and in some plant sources (e.g., walnuts and other tree nuts, flaxseed, and various vegetables). Monounsaturated fat is abundant in olive oil, nuts, and avocados. More than half the fat calories in a Mediterranean Diet come from monounsaturated fats (mainly from olive oil) rather than butter.

The diet is also high in foods like legumes, nuts, seeds, grains, poultry, and fish while low in red meat and dairy products. There is also moderate consumption of wine.

The Mediterranean Diet has attracted interest due to the traditionally lower rates of diet-related diseases (e.g., heart disease and cancer) within the region. But this may not be entirely due to the diet. Lifestyle factors (such as more physical activity and extended social support systems) may also play a part.

How it Works

The Mediterranean Diet has a relatively high fat intake (about 35 to 45% of daily calories, mostly in monounsaturated and polyunsaturated fats). As mentioned, the Mediterranean Diet is known for its use of olive oil as the principal fat, but also for its use of canola oil, which is rich in omega-3 fatty acids. Olive oil does not contain omega-3 fatty acids, but it does contain monounsaturated fats and may have beneficial effects such as improving insulin and blood glucose levels, and reducing blood pressure. The diet uses very little butter, margarine, or other fats, and no trans-fats or hydrogenated fats.

Although there are several variations of the Mediterranean Diet, there are some general characteristics, such as the following:

- The bulk of the diet comes from plant sources, including whole grains, breads, pasta, polenta (from corn), bulgur, couscous (from wheat), rice, potatoes, fruits, vegetables, legumes (beans and lentils), seeds, and nuts.

- There is high consumption of olive oil (emphasis on consuming monounsaturated fat).

- Fruits and vegetables are eaten in large quantities. They are usually fresh, unprocessed, grown locally, and consumed in season.

- Eggs are used sparingly—up to four eggs per week.

- There is moderate consumption of fish and poultry, which are consumed only one to three times per week (less than one pound per week combined), with fish preferred over poultry.

- Moderate consumption of wine (two to three times a week) is encouraged.

- Dairy products are consumed in small amounts daily, mainly as cheese and yogurt (one ounce of cheese and one cup of yogurt daily).

- Red meat is consumed only a few times per month (less than one pound per month total).

- Honey is the principal sweetener, and sweets are eaten only a few times per week.

Olive Oil

An important source of fat in the Mediterranean Diet is olive oil, which is used almost exclusively in cooking instead of butter, margarine, or other fats. Olive oil is a rich source of monounsaturated fat, which is protective against heart disease, possibly because it displaces saturated fat from the diet. Olive oil is also a source of antioxidants including vitamin E. It is important to remember that olive oil is used to prepare vegetable dishes, tomato sauces, and salads, and to fry fish.

Fruits and Vegetables

The Mediterranean Diet emphasizes food from plant sources, including fruits and vegetables, tomatoes, breads and grains, beans, nuts, and seeds. It also emphasizes a variety of minimally processed and, wherever possible, seasonally fresh and locally grown foods. You get to eat five or more servings of fresh fruits and vegetables, and six or more servings of whole grains and legumes.

Tomatoes, featured quite heavily in Mediterranean food, are a major source of antioxidants. Cooking, as in the preparation of tomato sauces, is recommended as it increases the availability of lycopene, one of the main antioxidants in tomatoes.

Fish

Fish is a staple of the Mediterranean Diet. In particular, oily fish such as sardines, have important health benefits. Oily fish, a source of omega-3 fatty acids, are particularly beneficial to heart health.

Wine

Throughout the Mediterranean, wine is drunk in moderation and usually taken with meals. For men moderation is two glasses per day, and for women usually one glass per day. Advocates of the Mediterranean Diet also contend that red wine is a significant factor in reducing heart disease.

Red wine contains a vast array of plant compounds with health-promoting qualities called phytonutrients. Among them, flavanoids, which are powerful antioxidants, protect against LDL-C oxidation.

Advantages

- This Mediterranean Diet has not only been proven to reduce the risk factors for heart disease but will also help prevent and control the ravages of all chronic illnesses including obesity, hypertension, diabetes, cancer, and inflammatory conditions.
- The Mediterranean Diet is not as restrictive as some of the other diets.
- This is not a weight loss diet; it is rather a health plan that will assist your body to reach and maintain its optimal weight.

Disadvantages

- Some dieters have complained it was hard to adapt to the Mediterranean Diet because it differed significantly from their usual dietary eating habits.

Summary

The Mediterranean Diet offers a healthy alternative for many Americans that consume far too much saturated fat, sodium, and processed foods. It is an ideal eating pattern for prevention of cardiovascular disease. The essence of this diet is the use of natural, whole foods and the avoidance of highly processed foods. The diet offers foods that are tasty, economical, and easy to prepare. Another benefit is that many people are more familiar with purchasing, preparing, and eating Mediterranean foods than some foods that are central to other dietary therapies. Several noted nutritionists and research projects have concluded that this diet is one of the most healthful in the world in terms of preventing such illnesses as heart disease and cancer, and increasing life expectancy.

Although olive oil is recommended it should be used as a substitute for other fats and is not used in addition to them. In other words, consumers may have to significantly reduce fat intake from meat and dairy products, margarine, cooking oils, and other sources. Wine is recommended with meals in the Mediterranean diet; those with health conditions and restrictions should use caution.

Dieticians have been quick to point out that there may be other factors that influence the effectiveness of the Mediterranean Diet. Getting plenty of physical exercise is important, as is reducing stress. They have also noted that the attitude toward eating and mealtimes may be a factor in their good health. Meals are regarded as important and joyful occasions and are shared with family and friends. In many Mediterranean countries, people generally take the time to relax after lunch, the largest meal of the day.

35

Negative Calorie Diet

Overview

The Negative Calorie Diet works on the premise that eating certain "negative calorie foods" (like an apple), allows you to lose weight. It works on the premise that negative calorie foods take up more caloric energy to digest than the calories that are in them. Your body has to expend energy in order to digest and absorb foods; in fact, 10% of your daily caloric intake is used to process foods in your body. As a result, your body is actually burning fat.

The negative calorie foods that are allowed in this diet include mainly vegetables and fruits such as asparagus, beets, onions, radishes, carrots, spinach, zucchini, broccoli, green cabbage, carrots, cauliflower, apples, oranges, pineapple, grapefruit, blueberries, papaya, cantaloupes, and cranberries. The surplus of vitamins stored in these foods will create a reaction in your digestive process that is said to lead to weight loss.

How it Works

For example if you eat an apple, which contains 50 calories, it would take a certain amount of energy for your body to process all of the nutrients and vitamins within the apple. In eating the apple, you would burn more than 50 calories; however, this is also highly dependent on the individual and their level of activity. Let's just say the net result is that you will burn 25 calories for every apple you eat. This is why advocates of the Negative Calorie Diet encourage you to eat frequent healthy meals, in doing so you are actually increasing the speed of your metabolism.

Advantages

- The Negative Calorie Diet is fairly straightforward.
- It promotes consumption of foods rich in vitamins and minerals.

- The diet increases the body's metabolism.

Disadvantages

- Following the Negative Calorie Diet may not be enough to create permanent and satisfactory weight loss.
- Because of the lack of scientific information in general regarding this diet, it seems to be more theoretical than practical.

Summary

The Negative Calorie Diet is controversial because the theory is not scientifically sound. No foods actually possess "negative calories". Critics purport that by following the Negative Calorie Diet you are potentially offsetting your positive calorie energy reserves, canceling out the effectiveness of weight training. The critics argue that we need calories to create energy both for exercise and for recovering from exercise. On the other side of the debate, advocates of the Negative Calorie Diet concede it is true that there are no foods that contain negative calories. However, they do argue that by eating certain foods you are increasing the metabolic processes, which can result in weight loss.

A better option for long-term weight loss success would be consuming such foods as part of a balanced diet with exercise. By doing this you have a better chance for long-term weight loss success.

36

NutriSystem Diet

Overview

NutriSystem started out as a weight loss center-based diet program, like Weight Watchers and Jenny Craig, but has now repositioned itself as an online weight-management program. The core of the plan relies on Nutri-System foods used as entrees for breakfast, lunch and dinner as well as snacks. You don't have to buy their prepackaged foods to participate in the program, but the NutriSystem meals revolve around the NuCrusine foods, making it difficult to follow the plan without buying the products. The entrees are also supplemented with fruits, vegetables, and skim milk.

All the meals and snacks fit into an easy-to-follow meal plan that stresses proper portions and eating six times a day to fuel your metabolism and keep you from feeling hungry. The meals are carefully calorie controlled so the dieter does not need to count calories in order to lose weight.

How it Works

The NutriSystem Diet is divided into two phases: weight loss, followed by weight maintenance. In the first phase, dieters eat NutriSystem prepackaged foods seven days a week and supplement these meals with fresh fruits, vegetables, and skim milk. The time spent on the reduced caloric diet depends on individual goal weights. The weight-maintenance program generally lasts up to one year, during which dieters eat NutriSystem foods two days a week and regular foods the other five days of the week.

There are more than 100 different prepackaged, shelf-stable, microwave-able NuCuisine entrees and snacks to choose from, including entrees that range from Tex-Mex Rice and Beans to Spicy Oriental Noodles with vegetables and peanuts, to old standbys like macaroni and cheese. Dieters can make their own menus from the prepackaged foods, or they can choose from diet meal packages suited to different tastes, such as Active Lifestyle, All-American, Healthy Lifestyles, International Light and Lean, and Traditional Favorites.

The meal plans are based on low-fat food choices from the USDA Food Guide Pyramid. Like Jenny Craig, the NutriSystem Diet consists of 20% protein, 20% fat, and 60% carbohydrates.

Membership in the online weight-loss community is free of charge. New members are assigned a personal weight-loss counselor, who will track their progress and offer advice. Members can make an appointment with their assigned counselor or log online anytime for help from any available counselor. New members will also receive a menu plan, a catalog of products, a good diary, a weight chart, and an online weekly newsletter. Members are also given the option of talking to "NutriBuddies," fellow NutriSystem dieters who offer support. Other services offered by NutriSystem include chat room support groups and a virtual exercise instructor that allows you to store your own customized exercise program.

Advantages

- The NutriSystem Diet emphasizes the role of regular exercise, provides a weekly newsletter and chat rooms, and includes a weekly one-on-one email chat with a personal counselor to help you stay on track.

- The meal plan is based on low-fat food choices from the Food Guide Pyramid and recommends a balanced diet that includes all types of foods.

- If you're the type of person who has trouble with meal planning and portion control, and doesn't want to think about food choices or even prepare meals that can't be microwaved, this plan may be for you.

- The diet can lead to weight loss at a rate of one or two pounds per week.

- The chat rooms and online counseling are helpful to dieters.

- NutriSystem's shift to an online dieting service offers more flexibility to people with irregular schedules and little free time to attend meetings.

Disadvantages

- The NutriSystem NuCuisine foods cost about $50 a week, so you need to examine your budget before signing on to the program.

- This plan works well if you're single or eat alone; however, if you have a family to cook for you'll either need to buy enough Nutri-System meals for everyone or prepare two separate meals.

- Once the diet program ends, you need to learn how to maintain your weight loss without the prepackaged foods. True, as you get closer to your goal, you are weaned off the NutriSystem Diet foods and you start making your own meals, but you must pay close attention to this part of the NutriSystem diet program in order to maintain your weight loss in the long term.

Summary

Overall, the NutriSystem Diet is a nutritionally sound, reduced-calorie diet. The diet was developed in accordance with weight-loss recommendations from the American Dietetic Association and the National Institutes of Health. This program is perfect for someone who likes structure and prepackaged convenience foods, and doesn't like to cook. However, anyone who craves the fresh taste of pan sautéed fish, roasted chicken, or a sizzling steak right off the grill isn't going to be won over by the taste of freeze-dried scrambled eggs.

Like the Jenny Craig Diet plan and other similar programs that offer pre-planned menus with packaged foods, nutritionists have reservations with the NutriSystem Diet. Dieters should be prepared to learn how to maintain weight loss by making the right food and cooking choices once the diet program is over.

37

Omega Diet

Overview

The Omega Diet, designed by Artemis Simopoulos, M.D. and Jo Robinson, as detailed in their book of the same name, is a solidly-based Mediterranean nutritional program that emphasizes the right balance of fatty acids along with choosing plenty of fruits and vegetables. The Omega Diet is also rich in grains, which are loaded with nutrients and antioxidants. According to Simopoulos, "We function best when we eat foods that are similar to those eaten by our remote ancestors—a diet including an abundance of antioxidant-rich fruits and vegetables and the proper balance of essential fatty acids." Simopoulos believes that the modern American diet contains far more omega-6 fatty acids than omega-3 fatty acids, and that the imbalance of these fats makes us more vulnerable to heart disease, cancer, obesity, inflammations, autoimmune disease, allergies, diabetes, and depression.

How it Works

Key to the Omega Diet are the omega-3 and omega-6 fatty acids, both of which are needed to stay healthy. Simopoulos maintains that in the right proportions, these fatty acids can do wonders for your cholesterol and blood pressure and help fight off cancer. Japanese, European, and Mediterranean diets typically have two-to-one ratios of omega-6 to omega-3 fatty acids, says Simopoulos. In the United States, the ratio of omega-6 to omega-3 fatty acids in diets is about 20 to 1—much too high for a healthy lifestyle, leaving Americans susceptible to heart disease, obesity, autoimmune diseases, and diabetes.

Omega-3 fatty acids can be found in a variety of foods, including cold-water fish, walnuts, dark green leafy vegetables, flaxseeds, and even enriched eggs. They can also be found in oils such as canola, walnut or flaxseed oil. Monounsaturated fats can be found in olives, avocados and nuts such as almonds, pecans, and peanuts. Omega-6 polyunsaturated fats are found primarily in safflower, sunflower, corn, cottonseed, and soybean oils. Most people consume too many omega-6 fatty acids. Fortunately, by consuming more omega-3 fatty acids, people can offset these risks.

Seven basic guidelines make up the Omega Diet:

1. Enrich your diet with omega-3 fatty acids found in fatty fish, walnuts, and green leafy vegetables.
2. Use monounsaturated oils such as olive or canola oil.
3. Eat seven or more servings of fruits and vegetables daily.
4. Eat more vegetable proteins such as peas, beans, and nuts.
5. Avoid saturated fat by choosing low-fat meat and dairy products.
6. Avoid oils high in omega-6 fatty acids, such as corn or soybean oils.
7. Eliminate the intake of trans-fatty acids by cutting back on margarine, vegetable shortening, and most prepared snacks and convenience foods.

It's important to note that increased fruit and vegetable consumption is vital to a healthy diet. While most health authorities, including the American Heart Association, are recommending five servings of fruits and vegetables, the Omega Diet encourages people to eat at least seven servings a day.

Advantages

- This Omega Diet has not only been proven to reduce the risk factors for heart disease but will also help prevent and control the ravages of all chronic illnesses including obesity, hypertension, diabetes, cancer, and inflammatory conditions.

- Omega-3 fatty acids may also be an important component in the development and maintenance of the central nervous system as well as stemming the effects of Alzheimer's and other diseases related to the nervous system.

Disadvantages

- Some dieters have complained that the Omega Diet was hard to adapt to because it differed significantly from their own dietary eating habits.

Summary

The Omega Diet offers a healthy alternative for many Americans that consume far too much saturated fat, sodium, and processed foods. It is an ideal eating pattern for prevention of cardiovascular disease. The essence of this diet is the use of natural, whole foods and the avoidance of highly processed ones. Nutritionists believe that current understanding and scientific evidence are adequate to recommend this diet widely as a practical, effective, and enjoyable strategy.

38

Peanut Butter Diet

Overview

The Peanut Butter Diet, a book by *Prevention* editor Holly McCord, is an ingenious blend of populist diet and scientific evidence. The diet is based on a small but growing body of research that indicates adding certain types of fat into the diet can actually help folks lose weight. Dietary fat actually promotes satiety, the feeling of satisfaction after a meal. Consequently, any diet that includes regular helpings of peanut butter (one of America's favorite comfort foods) is likely to leave dieters feeling less deprived and more willing to achieve their weight loss goals.

According to McCord, the diet takes off about half a pound a week, for a total of 25 pounds a year. The calorie allowance is 1,500 calories a day for women and 2,200 calories a day for men.

How it Works

In case you're thinking this diet sounds way too good to be true, in addition to monounsaturated fats, the other major food groups in the Peanut Butter Diet are vegetables, whole grains and potatoes, lean proteins, fruits and calcium-rich foods. It is also recommended that you get a fair amount of exercise—45 minutes of exercise each day.

The key to making this miracle work is portion control. The Peanut Butter Diet permits four (tablespoon-size) servings twice a day of peanut butter for women. Men are allotted six tablespoons of peanut butter twice a day. Don't exceed the recommended peanut butter servings given in the diet since two tablespoons of peanut butter contain 190 calories.

A typical menu for one day on the Peanut Butter Diet might be the following:

Breakfast

2 tablespoons of peanut butter; maple syrup waffles; one cup of fat-free milk, plain or in cafe latte.

Lunch

Tuna Salad: three ounces of drained, water-packed, white albacore tuna with two teaspoons of reduced-calorie mayonnaise, one-half teaspoon of Dijon mustard, and two tablespoons of finely chopped carrots and celery. One and one-half cups of baby carrots red bell pepper strips, three-quarters of a cup of calcium-enriched V-8 juice, and of course, two tablespoons of peanut butter.

Snack

Two tablespoons of peanut butter, one cup of celery sticks, six-ounce can of calcium-enriched V-8 juice

Dinner

Tahitian chicken with peanut butter mango sauce served over one-half cup of cooked brown basmati rice, one-half cup of cooked spinach.

Evening Treat

Orange, pear, or other fruit of your choice

Advantages

- The Peanut Butter Diet is easy to follow.
- Typically dieters on high-fat diets stay on their diet longer and keep the weight off, as opposed to dieters on low-fat, high-carbohydrate diets.
- In a nutshell it's no more than a slow weight-loss plan, with a few extra calories and regular servings of peanut butter.
- When compared to other diets, the peanut butter diet appears less demanding in terms of do's and don'ts.

Disadvantages

- The Peanut Butter Diet isn't suitable for those with peanut allergies.
- Some dieters simply get tired of eating peanut butter on a daily basis.

Summary

The Peanut Butter Diet is no more than a slow-weight-loss plan, with a few extra calories and regular servings of peanut butter. It's true that peanut butter is high in fat but most of it is monounsaturated, the same "good fat" that's found in olive oil. Studies have shown a diet high in monounsaturated fat from peanuts and peanut butter can actually lower your risks for heart disease and diabetes—perhaps even better than the low-fat, high-carbohydrate diets. Diets high in peanuts and rich in monounsaturated fat are just as good at lowering total cholesterol and bad LDL cholesterol as very low fat diets.

People who eat a diet high in foods like olive oil, avocados, and peanut butter are more likely to lose weight and keep it off than people following a more regimented, lower-fat diet. Nutritionists suggest dieters feel fuller and eat less after snacking on peanut butter than after eating other foods.

Perricone Diet

Overview

The Perricone Diet is not so much about losing weight as it is about improving nutrition in order to reduce damage to the outer layers of your skin caused by free radicals. Touted as "the wrinkle cure," this diet, devised by dermatologist Nicholas Perricone M.D., assumes that eating a diet rich in anti-aging, anti-oxidants will reduce inflammatory changes in the body and thereby prevent wrinkles. By choosing the right foods such as avocados, berries, dark green leafy vegetables, and salmon, Perricone promises that your skin will look younger and healthier. Perricone believes that sugar and foods with a high glycemic index such as bread, bagels, bananas, pizza, pasta, and potatoes lead to the inflammation that is at the root of wrinkles and aging skin.

How it Works

The basis of the diet is a 28-day program that aims to reduce saturated fats, refined sugars, and other high glycemic carbohydrates.

Whole grains, legumes/beans, and non-instant oatmeal are preferred. Avoid all refined carbohydrates and foods rated greater than 50 on the glycemic index. Carbohydrates that have a low glycemic index are preferred since they break down slowly and their glucose is gradually released into the bloodstream. Perricone believes that if your blood sugar rises too quickly, inflammatory chemicals that contribute to the aging process will be released. Too much sugar equals sagging, wrinkled skin.

Perricone recommends eating fish (especially wild salmon, or canned Alaskan red/pink salmon) as well as egg whites, skinless chicken, and turkey breast. Salmon is strongly recommended because it contains high amounts of protein, a coenzyme Q-10, which is a powerful antioxidant, plus it's rich in dimethylaminoethanol (DMAE). According to Perricone, DMAE increases tone in the skin. The salmon should be wild, or at the least organic.

Besides fish (or other lean proteins such as chicken), the Perricone Diet calls for small amounts of fat from olive oil, or nuts and lots of fruits and vegetables such as avocados, bell peppers, berries, cantaloupe/honeydew melons, dark leafy green vegetables (spinach, kale), orange-colored squash, and tomatoes. Perricone recommends not eating dried fruits.

Perricone advocates reducing saturated fats and avoiding trans-fatty acids (a.k.a. hydrogenated fats). Instead, use extra virgin olive oil, (rich in oleic acid which helps omega-3 fatty acids to protect cells).

Substitute green tea for coffee, which contains catechin polyphenols—anti-oxidants that boost metabolism and slow aging. Green tea can also block the absorption of bad fats by 30 percent, while the amino acid theonine promotes a sense of calm and improves your mood. The diet discourages drinking coffee because coffee is acidic and dehydrates your skin. Other drinks discouraged include diet soda because it has too many chemicals; fruit juice, which is filled with sugar and can be acidic; and alcohol, which dehydrates your skin. Perricone strongly recommends drinking plenty of spring water (8–10 glasses), which is great for the skin. Water adds elasticity to your skin and flushes impurities from your body. The drinking of milk should be limited.

The Perricone Diet recommends taking nutrient supplements including alpha lipoic acid, vitamins A, B1, B2, B3, B5, B6, B12, folate, biotin, vitamin C, vitamin C ester, vitamin E, calcium, chromium, magnesium, selenium, l-carnitine, acetyl l-carnitine, coenzyme Q10, l-glutamine, omega-3 fatty acids, grape seed extract, gamma linoleic acid, and turmeric.

Skin treatments are also recommended such as sunscreens, cleansers, moisturizers, eye-care products and enriched night cream and creams with ingredients such as vitamin C, vitamin C ester, alpha lipoic acid, DMAE, PPC, tocotrienol, and olive oil.

Advantages

- The Perricone Diet contains numerous antioxidants believed to promote overall health.
- The benefits of the Perricone Diet are better skin, fewer aging effects, and better protection against a host of diseases and conditions.

Disadvantages

- The Perricone Diet limits food choices. For example, you've got to like eating salmon, since eating it is an almost daily ritual on this plan.
- Eating wild salmon on a regular basis can be pricey.
- The nutritional supplements and skin care products that Perricone markets are very high-priced.

Summary

The Perricone Diet program is a reasonably healthy eating plan in spite of its restrictions of certain foods—never mind the anti-aging benefits. Even so, except for his commendation of salmon, his emphasis on fish, low-GI carbohydrates, olive oil, fruits, and vegetables is a step in the right direction.

40

Pritikin Diet

Overview

The Pritikin Diet was developed by Nathan Pritikin, founder of the Pritikin Longevity Center in California, as an attempt to markedly reduce the risk of heart disease. Although not principally a weight loss diet, many people who follow the Pritikin Diet tend to lose weight.

The Pritikin Diet is a low-fat, high-carbohydrate eating plan. It focuses on complex carbohydrates, fresh fruits, and vegetables eaten raw or cooked. It is high in fiber, low in cholesterol, and extremely low in saturated fat and total fat, containing less than 10% of total daily calories from fat. The consumption of seafood, rich in omega-3 fatty acids, is encouraged, followed by skinless chicken, and lean red meat.

Processed foods such as pasta and white bread, animal proteins, eggs, and most types of fats are eliminated in favor of whole grains, fruits, and vegetables. Severe restrictions are placed on refined sweets.

How it Works

While the Pritikin Diet doesn't have you counting calories, it does require calculating the average caloric density of each meal, which is done by combining the different caloric food groups. The basic idea is to fill up on low-caloric and medium-caloric density foods that have relatively few calories per pound, such as apples and oatmeal with only occasional forays into high-caloric density foods. The higher the caloric density of any given food, the more likely it is to cause weight gain. Corn, for instance, starts out at a somewhat reasonable 490 calories per pound, but chocolate chip cookies skyrocket to 2,140 calories per pound.

The Pritikin Diet provides menu examples and general dietary suggestions that emphasize eating whole, unprocessed foods like fruits, vegetables, and low-fat carbohydrate foods. This emphasis on complex carbohydrates makes it high in vitamins, minerals, and fiber, and low in sodium. In short, it encompasses a very healthy range of foods and generous portions, which should fill you up without any danger of weight gain.

A typical breakfast includes a bowl of hot grain cereal, bananas and blueberries, half a grapefruit, skim milk, and a cup of green tea. Lunch might include a hearty bean and vegetable soup, large mixed raw salad with oil-free dressing, crusty whole meal bread or crackers, an ear of corn, and fresh fruit or herbal tea or mineral water. A typical dinner could include poached salmon, steamed vegetables, brown rice, green salad with balsamic vinegar, and a glass of wine or herbal tea. Snacks throughout the day would include bread or rice crackers, fresh vegetables (carrot and celery sticks), and fat-free plain yogurt mixed with fresh fruit.

In addition to eating three meals a day, the Pritikin Diet encourages snacking between meals. Good snack choices include low-fat, high-fiber soups like minestrone and other bean based varieties, whole fruits, vegetables, and salads. Pritikin believes eating frequently, which keeps you from being hungry, prevents the triggering of your fat instinct, and keeps your body burning fat.

The Pritikin Diet recommends regular exercise, such as walking for at least 45 minutes each day averaging 12 to 15 miles a week.

Advantages

- The Pritikin Diet is good for those folks with a family history of heart disease.

- It encourages eating balanced meals that include high-fiber fruits, vegetables, beans, and grains.

- A large body of scientific literature demonstrates the benefits of a low-fat, high-fiber diet in the prevention of many degenerative diseases, including cancer and heart disease.

- The Pritikin Diet also encourages daily exercise and stress-reduction techniques.

- The Pritikin Diet can lead to weight loss.

- This diet is perfect for those who don't like calorie counting or watching portions. So, there is a better chance for people to stay with the diet.
- Meals are customized to meet personal needs and tastes from a wide range of foods and menus.
- The diet can lower cholesterol and triglyceride levels.

Disadvantages

- The Pritikin Diet is difficult for many people because they have to give up animal products and dairy products.
- Most dieters may have a difficult time sticking to this diet with its low daily intake of fat at 10%.
- In spite of the focus on eating more whole foods, the plan is low in several nutrients, including zinc, iron, calcium, folate, and the B vitamins—particularly vitamin B12—which are found naturally only in animal foods.
- Many medical and nutrition professionals agree with this plant-based, high-fiber approach. However, they believe that a 10% total daily fat intake is too low. Dietary fat provides essential fatty acids and the fat-soluble vitamins A, D, E, and K needed for normal cell function and tissue growth.
- Low-fat diets often increase hunger, leading to overeating. When you significantly decrease the fat in your diet, your body will start craving calories from sugars and carbohydrates.
- There is no specific diet plan. Each dieter must design their meals by following Pritikin's general dietary advice.

Summary

There seems to be little dispute that you will lose weight with this diet. However, the extremely low fat content of this diet (10% of total calories) will make those following it often feel hungry resulting in the likelihood the weight will return after one stops strictly adhering to the diet.

Another problem is that the fat content being so low may be harmful to our health. Because dietary fat is so severely restricted, Pritikin dieters may not be able to consume a sufficient amount of the healthy fats, especially the omega-3 fats. In addition, absorption of the fat-soluble vitamins (A, D, E, and K) may be impaired with such low intakes of dietary fat.

The typical American diet averages between 35 and 45% fat. The Dietary Guidelines for Americans recommends a diet with approximately 30% of total calories coming from fat.

41

Protein Power Diet

Overview

The ideas behind the Protein Power Diet were originally published in a book titled *Protein Power* (1996) authored by Drs. Michael and Mary Eades. The Protein Power Diet is similar in many ways to the Atkins Diet. The premise behind the Protein Power Diet is to reduce the intake of carbohydrates, which will reduce the amount of insulin released in the body. High insulin levels, they say, not only leads to weight gain and obesity but can cause health problems such as heart disease, high cholesterol, hypertension, fluid retention, and diabetes. By reducing the carbohydrate intake while keeping protein intake high, your body switches over to using fat for fuel.

The biggest difference between the Protein Power Diet and the Atkins Diet is the way caloric values are determined. On the Atkins Diet, as long as you don't exceed your daily carbohydrate intake, you can eat whatever and whenever you want. On the Protein Power Diet plan, your daily caloric intake is directly tied to your protein requirement.

How it Works

This plan begins with calculating your protein requirements, which are typically determined by analyzing the activity level of the individual in question. Active individuals may require as much as one gram of protein per pound of lean body mass, while 0.5 gram of protein per pound of lean body mass will suffice for inactive people. The lean body mass is calculated using standardized charts that use height, hip, and abdomen measurements in women, and weight, wrist, and waist measurements in men. Incidentally, this is the same formula for protein requirements as used in the Zone Diet.) Dieters are advised to eat the minimum amounts of protein based on the above calculations, but are told they can eat more if they are hungry. People on this diet may also want to invest in protein supplements.

People on this diet are only allowed to eat between 30 and 50 grams of carbohydrates per day depending on their activity level. Phase 1 of this diet is for those that are 20% or more over their ideal body weight. These dieters reduce carbohydrate intake to a maximum of 30 grams per day. Phase 2 of the diet is for those less than 20% over their ideal body weight, and requires a reduction to 50 grams a day of carbohydrates. You need to count everything you consume while on this diet, and eat foods at specific times.

Foods that you are allowed to eat are all types of beef, pork, chicken, turkey, wild game, eggs, many non-starchy vegetables (except carrots), very small portions of fruits (except bananas), and very small amounts of dairy products, whole grain products, and dried beans.

Advantages

- The primary benefit of the Protein Power Diet is rapid and substantial weight loss. Initially much of the weight loss is due to water loss, but long-term weight loss occurs due to a low carbohydrate intake with the body burning stored fat for energy.

- Because you can eat as much as you like of the permitted foods, you don't get hungry.

- It is argued that a low carbohydrate diet is more natural for the human body because grains in the form of wheat and rice only became a regular part of our diet 10,000 years ago so our bodies have not had time to evolve to cope with these grains satisfactorily.

- Some research indicates that people with Type 2 diabetes have better insulin function and better blood sugar control on a low carbohydrate diet.

- It is considered to lower risk for chronic illnesses, like heart disease, high blood pressure, and diabetes

- Good for managing many health disorders including headaches, blood sugar disorders, food intolerances, allergies, and many other health problems.

Disadvantages

- One of the major drawbacks of the Protein Power Diet involves estimating how many carbohydrates to eat in a day. This is quite hard, if not impossible.

- Any diet that limits carbohydrates causes the body to rely on fat or muscle for energy. When our body breaks down stored fat to supply energy, a byproduct called ketones are formed. Ketones suppress appetite, but they also cause fatigue, nausea, and a potentially dangerous fluid loss. In sever cases it can cause unconsciousness, and even lead to a coma. Anyone with diabetes, or heart or kidney problems should NOT follow a diet that promotes the formation of ketones, including the Atkins Diet.

- People with diabetes taking insulin are at risk of becoming hypoglycemic if they do not eat appropriate carbohydrates.

- People who exercise regularly may experience low energy levels and muscle fatigue from low carbohydrate intake.

- The Protein Power Diet is not recommended for pregnant women or nursing mothers, or for people being treated for high blood pressure.

- Eating unlimited amounts of fat, especially saturated fat found in meat products, can lead to increased risk of heart disease in the long term.

- The Protein Power Diet doesn't conform to the American Heart Association's dietary guidelines for a healthy heart.

- Adherence to the Protein Power Diet can result in vitamin and mineral deficiencies such as vitamin B, calcium, and potassium.

- Restricting carbohydrates means eating a low-fiber diet, which can cause constipation.

- The diet lacks phytochemicals derived from carbohydrate-rich plant foods, which are important cancer-fighting agents.

- The Protein Power Diet may not always be easy to follow because it is somewhat restrictive in the nature of the carbohydrate foods you can eat.

- If you go back to a higher carbohydrate diet again, the pounds will return.

- Studies show that restrictive diets, which eliminate several foods or food groups, have the highest failure rates over time—a pretty dismal outlook.

- One unattractive feature is that the diet can also cause bad breath. This is a result of ketosis—the state the body goes into during starvation.

- This is a difficult program to follow long-term for those who enjoy eating sweets, breads, fruits, or other carbohydrate-containing foods

Summary

Using the Protein Power Diet for a limited time for weight loss should not cause any major problems; however, its design is not ideal for long-term use because of a number of weaknesses. First, estimating protein needs on the basis of activity level is not supported by known medical research. Second, as with all low-carbohydrate diets, the Protein Power Diet can cause ketosis, which may produce some health hazards in a long-term eating plan. Third, the idea that a high-protein, low-carbohydrate diet helps you lose weight by reducing insulin levels is inaccurate. Scientific research shows being overweight is not a result of insulin levels being high, but that being overweight causes insulin problems. Reducing your intake of any food will achieve this.

Finally, the Eades emphatically state that resistance training (lifting weights) is "better" than aerobic activity. No reliable science suggests one of these two forms of exercise is superior—both are equally important for overall fitness and weight management.

42

Raw Food Diet

Overview

The Raw Food Diet—often called a Living Food Diet—is based on consuming unprocessed, preferably organic, whole plant-based foods, of which most should be uncooked. The Raw Food Diet has been around since the 1950s, when Ann Wigmore, a self-taught nutritionist, advocated the belief that a diet of raw fruits and vegetables could cure various diseases. The Raw Food Diet continued to exist as a radical offshoot of the vegetarian diet until 1975, when computer programmer-turned-nutritionist Viktoras Kulvinskas published *Survival into the 21st Century*. The book is considered to be the first modern publication that deals with the Raw Food Diet. But the diet really didn't take off until the late 1990s, when high-powered chefs and celebrities rediscovered the diet and began singing its praises.

A typical Raw Food Diet may consist of a least 75% raw food, although there are stricter versions that insist on no cooking and a 100% vegetarian dietary regimen. Where cooking is allowed, it is usually to permit the addition of some cooked whole grains and pulses, plus good quality fish and lean poultry.

Raw Food Diet practitioners eat fruits and vegetables (organic whenever possible), nuts, sprouted seeds, legumes, and a heavy dose of herbs and spices. Even canned fruits and vegetables are avoided because of the way they are processed.

Followers who subscribe to the Raw Food Diet claim that all raw foods contain essential food enzymes, which are fundamental to human health. The cooking process (i.e., heating foods above 116°F) is thought to destroy food enzymes as well as vitamins, minerals, and protein. These believers also claim that cooking food renders it toxic and is the major cause of health problems. Plus cooking is believed to destroy the food's energy field. The intensity of beliefs held by raw food proponents vary with each individual, yet they all support the ideology that cooking is an unnatural process that destroys important and vital nutrients in foods.

How it Works

First, fruits and vegetables are not usually eaten at the same time when raw because they don't digest the same. Typically people who eat raw food for a significant length of time eat fruit in the mornings and vegetables the rest of the day.

Preparation of raw food recipes usually calls for a blender, a food processor, a juicer, and a dehydrator. People who follow the Raw Food Diet use particular techniques to prepare foods. These include sprouting seeds, grains and beans; soaking nuts and dried fruits; and juicing fruits and vegetables. The only cooking that is allowed is via a dehydrator. This piece of equipment blows hot air through the food but never reaches a temperature higher than 116°F.

Some of the more popular foods are fresh fruits and vegetables, nuts, seeds, beans, grains, legumes, dried fruits, seaweeds, sun-dried fruits, other organic or natural foods that have not been processed, freshly made fruit and vegetable juices, purified water (not tap), and milk from a young coconut.

Advantages

- The Raw Food Diet is good for losing weight.
- Opponents of the diet believe it increases your energy levels.
- Following the diet improves the appearance of the skin.
- Raw food diets improve digestion.
- There is reduced risk of heart disease and certain cancers.

Disadvantages

- The Raw Food Diet is a very hard diet to maintain, long term.
- It is difficult to feed a whole family with such an uncompromising diet plan.
- It is not easy to design a proper balanced raw foods diet.

- The Raw Food Diet lacks the recommended amounts of several important vitamins and nutrients, including vitamin B12, calcium, and protein. When followed for an extended period of time, the diet can lead to severe nutritional deficiency.

- The diet may include occasional headaches, nausea, and mild depression.

- There is clearly a safety issue surrounding these raw foods, in that they must be free of harmful bacteria that typical sterilizing processes—such as cooking—would normally kill.

- The diet can be costly because the program advocates buying the pricier organic fruits and vegetables, and bottled water, to avoid pesticides.

- Food preparation—particularly without a blender, juicer, or high-powered mixer—can be time-consuming and arduous because most raw food recipes demand cutting, chopping, and blending of fruits, vegetables, and nuts.

Summary

While nutritionists have little problem with people eating raw foods (as long as they're clean), many are dubious about basing an entire diet on the concept. It's true that the Raw Food Diet is nutrient dense and there is little or no saturated fat, and it is low in sodium, high in potassium, and fiber-rich. These factors are important in weight control and helping to reduce the risk of certain diseases, such as heart disease and some cancers.

However, eating only raw foods can considerably limit the variety of foods that can be included in the diet, such as meat, potatoes, and cereal products, which in turn can limit our nutrient intake. This could lead to nutritional deficiencies—in iron and calcium, for example—if followed for any length of time.

Proponents of the Raw Food Diet believe the cooking process destroys enzymes, vitamins, minerals and protein. In the diet's defense, cooking certain foods does reduce the vitamin content, but there are some beneficial compounds that are enhanced when they are cooked. Some studies also suggest that cooked tomatoes release more phytonutrients than raw ones. Also the lycopene found in tomatoes is a strong antioxidant linked to preventing several different diseases—and it's released with heat.

Proponents also believe that some enzymes are inactivated when food is heated, but this is not considered important because the body relies on its own enzymes for digestion.

Medical professionals take issue with claims that certain chronic diseases can be treated by eating raw food. Some people will accept that as truth and delay seeking appropriate diagnosis and treatment, and that could seriously impact long-term well-being of the dieter.

Another concern about the Raw Food Diet is the safety risks. Foods such as un-pasteurized milk and juice can harbor harmful bacteria, as can raw salad greens such as lettuce and spinach. Most foods in the Raw Food Diet are simple to prepare, and can be eaten immediately. However, other foods can require hours, or even days, of preparation to make the food palatable. Rice, for example, must be soaked in water for more than a day to soften it. Depending on the recipe, some food may also need to be dehydrated. This process, which emulates cooked food, can take days.

43

Revival Soy Diet

Overview

The Revival Soy Diet, developed by Dr. Aaron T. Tabor, is not necessarily a weight-loss diet but more of a natural approach for effective relief of menopause symptoms, including hot flashes and night sweats. Tabor investigated numerous medical studies, which indicated significantly lower rates of menopause discomfort among Asian women when compared to women in the United States. Soy contains phytochemicals called isoflavones (pronounced i-so-flay-vones), which act like natural estrogens within the body.

It was later found that consumption of soy protein helps one lose weight. Soy protein is a low-fat source of high-quality protein (compared to many other protein sources) that can help you build lean muscle mass. Soy protein is also good at controlling insulin levels. Reduced insulin fluctuations result in fewer "sugar cravings." When combined with exercise and a healthy diet, soy protein makes an excellent "partner" in a successful weight loss plan.

How it Works

The Revival Soy Diet is based on using *Revival Soy* products as a dietary food supplement or in conjunction with other diet plans—including the popular low-carbohydrate diets. The company recommends following a number of simple rules to achieve long-term weight loss.

- Consume a Revival Soy bar or shake as a meal substitute one to two times per day.
- Take multivitamins every day.
- Reduce your intake of refined, simple carbohydrates like sweets, soda, white breads, and alcohol.
- Increase your intake of fruits and vegetables.
- Load up on foods naturally high in fiber, such as fruits, vegetables, legumes, and whole grains.

- Limit portions of foods in fat such as diary products, red meat, cakes, and pastries.

- Exercise at least three times a week for 20 minutes.

- Eat smaller portion sizes and eat more slowly.

- Drink a minimum of six full glasses of ice-cold water or other low- or no-calorie liquid per day.

- Find a "weight loss buddy" for emotional support and praise.

Advantages

- Scientific studies show that soy protein can help decrease body fat and increase lean body mass.

- Soy protein can also help decrease risk of cardiovascular disease.

- Soy protein is also a great source of energy and supports bone, breast and prostate health.

- Soy protein helps you feel fuller longer.

Disadvantages

- One Revival Soy shake is equal to six servings of soy foods, so there is a potential in consuming too much soy protein if you use more than two of their products per day.

Summary

Soy protein shakes and snacks have become a popular weight loss alternative. The conventional wisdom is that soy protein is healthy and effective in weight loss, lowering cholesterol, and minimizing menopause discomfort. Shakes and snacks can be an effective and convenient way of adding soy protein to your diet during your busy day. However, nutritionists point out that bars and shakes can never provide all the benefits of real food—so use caution when thinking long-term.

44

Richard Simmons Diet

Overview

Richard Simmons is an icon of the weight loss business, and has created a weight-loss empire by marketing everything from diet plans to videos to a variety of weight-loss supplements. Simmons diet plans are well rounded, and can give you the necessary motivation should you falter in your goals. His diet plans are updated regularly and repackaged to provide a variety of choices with lots of motivation and fun ways to add exercise to your life. Simmons places an enormous emphasis on physical activity, and this is the one trait of his weight-loss programs that stands out and puts it a notch above the rest. In fact, Richard Simmons was, and probably still is, best known for his exercise videos that emphasize aerobic activity to the beat of a wide variety of music, from disco to Broadway.

How it Works

The original diet program developed by Simmons was the Deal-A-Meal diet program. With the Deal-A-Meal program dieters kept track of the foods they ate by moving "cards" from one side of a wallet to the other after each meal. After all of the cards (representing food items) were moved from one side to the other, a dieter was done eating for the day.

Another diet program developed by Simmons' similar to Deal-A-Meal, is called the FoodMover. The FoodMover is different from Deal-A-Meal because it is a hand-held mini-computer with little windows that the dieter closes once a goal is reached or the food has been consumed. The device also has check boxes for exercise, vitamins, and Simmons' own motivational anecdotes.

The latest diet plan is called "Richard Simmons' Lose Weight and Celebrate." This Lose Weight and Celebrate program lays out a well-balanced and varied diet that admirably includes a minimum of seven servings of fruits and vegetables and two servings of low fat dairy foods a day. He also wisely recommends not going below 1,200 calories and drinking eight glasses of water each day. It's a no-nonsense program that sets clear guidelines but leaves individual food choices up to the dieter. There are no prepackaged foods, and he encourages you to choose from fresh foods like fish, strawberries, greens, oranges, and whole-grain breads. The foods are grouped according to categories, and the diet is set up much like the exchange system used for diabetics. For example, one slice of bread equals one bread exchange, eight ounces of skim milk equals one milk exchange, etc. You're allowed a certain number of exchanges from each group, depending on your daily calorie quota.

Advantages

- Simmons diet plans are considered balanced.
- Severely overweight dieters can begin to lose weight without having to give up the foods they love (and are actually addicted to).
- Simmons diet plans are easy to follow.
- Simmons offers an online support community.

Disadvantages

- Simmons diet plans can be costly.
- This is a hyper-commercial weight loss operation offering a bewildering array of weight loss products, supplements, and vitamins, including exercise videos, motivational cassettes, a small cookbook, and a dietary instruction booklet.
- Web site product pricing is not always clear.
- These programs are only good for severely overweight people.
- A serious diet will still be necessary after a severely overweight person is done using the Deal-A-Meal or FoodMover diet programs.

Summary

The Richard Simmons Diet plans are helpful because he acknowledges and accommodates the needs of even the most overweight people, despite his commercialism. The exchange lists and the meal plan will provide you with a great variety of food choices, and they will help you to control the distribution of calories, carbohydrate, protein, and fat throughout the day so that your meals can be balanced. Few nutritionists take any real issue with his diet programs, with the exception of the including and marketing of his own brand of supplements. If you follow his recommended calorie intakes, you should expect to lose about one to two pounds per week. It is a diet and exercise plan that's designed for the long haul and for long-term success.

Alternative diet programs for severely overweight dieters include Jenny Craig and Weight Watchers. Although a sensible and well-balanced diet consisting of fresh fruits, vegetables, and high quality protein sources would be even better.

45

Rosedale Diet

Overview

The Rosedale Diet, written by Dr. Ron Rosedale, could be described as a high fat, very low carbohydrate, low-protein diet. It is similar to the South Beach Diet and the Hamptons Diet (and even the Atkins Diet), yet places more emphasis on eating a lot more fat. The Rosedale Diet is based on the consumption of foods that are high in good fats such as omega-3 fatty acids.

The premise behind the Rosedale Diet is not focusing fat grams, carbohydrates, or calories like most diets but controlling the hormone leptin, a protein that is secreted by fat. Recent research has shown leptin tells your brain when to eat, how much to eat and, most importantly, when to stop eating. Rosedale says keeping this hormone down to the optimal low levels alerts the body that you've eaten enough and stored enough fat and need to burn off excess fat.

How it Works

The essence of the diet plan is a three-week phase where certain carbohydrates are reduced or eliminated. After the first three weeks, some of those foods can be eaten, but only in restricted amounts.

There are certain fruits and vegetables that must be avoided altogether such as bananas, cantaloupe, dried fruit (all varieties), grapes, honeydew, oranges, pineapple, watermelon, yams, pumpkin, white potatoes, and corn.

Rosedale recommends only 15 minutes of exercise daily.

Advantages

- The Rosedale Diet claims that dieters will permanently lose weight by controlling leptin.

Disadvantages

- The Rosedale Diet recommends supplements. This is not to say that all supplements are bad but they can be quite costly and probably wouldn't be necessary if you were eating a balanced diet.
- The only carbohydrates the author recommends are fibrous carbohydrates such as green vegetables. Starchy carbohydrates and grains are completely out.
- The diet recommends very little exercise.

Summary

The Rosedale Diet, despite containing a lot of (apparent) science, has very little that is new—it is certainly not the "breakthrough" that the author is claiming. The diet encourages dieters to shift to a more balanced range of foods including monounsaturated fats, complex carbohydrates, and no processed foods, which is a step in the right direction. However, nutritionists believe it cuts way back on healthful foods like fruits, vegetables and dairy. On the flip side, unlike other low-carbohydrate diets that encourage the widespread consumption of saturated fats, the Rosedale Diet places a lot of emphasis on consuming the right kind of fats—specifically, monounsaturated fats.

46

Rotation Diet

Overview

The Rotation Diet, developed by Dr. Martin Katahn, requires dieters to follow a diet for three weeks at a time, and then rotate off the diet for a short period and return to normal eating habits. The rotation theory is based on the belief that the majority of diets routinely fail because people tire of eating the same, boring foods, and because metabolism gradually slows during any diet that strictly limits calories.

How it Works

While on the Rotation Diet, you alternate your calorie intake over a three-week period in order to achieve a dramatic, quick weight loss. Women use a mixed diet consisting of a wide variety of foods, rotating from 600, to 900, and then to 1,200 calories a day over the three-week period. Men rotate from 1,200, to 1,500, to 1,800 calories a day over the course of the three weeks. After three weeks of dieting you rotate off the diet. During the maintenance period dieters are encouraged to gradually increase their intake of calories until they reach a point where they can eat and not regain any weight. After a one- to four-week break, dieters can follow another three-week rotation if they need to lose more weight. The strategy here is to avoid long stretches of low-calorie eating, which often cause your metabolism to slow down.

The basic plan calls for dieters to eat less fat and more fish, and walk or incorporate exercise into their daily routine.

Advantages

- The Rotation Diet claims that dieters will permanently lose weight because it will keep their metabolism at a consistent level to avoid regaining weight.

- This diet is set up so that you can go on and off the diet without having any negative repercussions.

Disadvantages

- Dieters may experience a few minor side effects while on the Rotation Diet such as fatigue, constipation, nausea, and diarrhea.
- There are other more serious side effects with this sort of rapid weight loss regimen, including the development of gallstones.
- To be healthy, we need a balance of foods from different food groups. It's quite difficult to get good nutrition in as few as 600 calories, especially if one eats the same foods day after day.

Summary

The Rotation Diet goes against mainstream nutritional recommendations when it says you can go off the diet when you reach your desired weight and that it shouldn't become a way of life. Nutritionists say the key to long-term weight loss is adopting real-life strategies for healthy eating and exercise habits that you can maintain over a lifetime. Going on and off a diet can lead to rebound binge eating and to gaining back more weight than was lost.

Critics also argue the daily caloric intakes are in many cases too low to meet energy needs thus resulting in fatigue, constipation, nausea, and diarrhea.

The diet also downplays the importance of exercise. Nutritionists maintain that for sustained weight loss, the best diet is usually a balanced diet with foods from all the nutritional food groups, which offers realistic weight reduction goals and provides a manageable eating plan. For most people, purely focusing on food is the problem in the first place, regardless of whether the food was healthy or unhealthy. Exercise is the one thing in common with all those who lose weight and keep it off.

47

Scan Diet

Overview

The Scan Diet, developed by a Scandinavian doctor, is based around eating lots of soy-based, nutrient-fortified meal replacement drinks. The diet allows for different amounts of calories a day depending on the needs of the person.

How it Works

There are three variants of the Scan Diet: the Attack Plan, the Balance Plan, and the Control Plan. A physician consultation is recommended before you start.

Attack Plan – Short-period weight loss (1,200 calories per day) to reduce weight quickly.

Balance Plan – Steady weight loss (1,500 calories per day) to lose weight steadily.

Control Plan – Long-term maintenance (1,800 calories per day) to maintain your weight long term.

The Attack Plan allows for safe weight reduction by replacing meals with five Scan diet servings each day, in addition to four servings of fruit and four servings of vegetables.

The Balance Plan, for continued, steady weight loss, calls for three Scan Diet servings, three servings of fruit, four servings of vegetables, and two well-balanced, low fat meals each day. The meals can include lean meat, bread, and pasta.

The Control Plan is designed for long-term weight maintenance. It calls for one Scan diet serving each day, plus three meals and snacks, including four servings of fruit and four servings of vegetables.

Advantages

- The Scan Diet is easy to follow.
- The diet does not stoop to unhealthy calorie levels, if dieters eat the additional food and don't just rely on the Scan meal replacements.
- The Scan Diet weans dieters off meal replacements and gradually introduces more healthful foods.
- The plan encourages at least 10 glasses of non-caffeinated, nonalcoholic beverages daily and 30 to 40 minutes of exercise three to four times a week.
- The diet may help lower cholesterol levels since one packet contains 18 grams of soy protein plus seven grams of soy fiber.

Disadvantages

- The Scan Diet plan never weans dieters off meal replacements entirely.
- The calorie levels in all three phases are pre-established, with little individual variation for age, activity, gender, or body composition.
- A diet of powdered meal-replacements does not seem like a long-term solution to weight loss.
- The high soy content may be a concern for women with a history of breast cancer, since many experts caution women at risk of breast cancer to limit soy intake, fearing the estrogen-like phytoestrogens it contains might actually fuel cancer cells.
- At $300 per month for the quick weight loss plan, it's expensive.
- The diet program doesn't teach you how to eat properly.
- It's not a good diet plan for families.

Summary

The Scan Diet appears to be safer and more nutritionally sound than past low-calorie liquid diets. However, it may not lead to permanent weight loss because it doesn't alter your eating habits in the long term. Like all meal-replacement diets, the big question about the Scan Diet is whether the weight loss benefits are sustainable when you leave the diet and start cooking and preparing meals for yourself. Still, for people who need help getting started, the Scan Diet may be one answer, especially if aided by the fine-tuning of a qualified nutritionist.

48

Scarsdale Diet

Overview

The Scarsdale Diet, developed by Dr. Herman Tarnower was a very popular diet in the 1970s. The diet is high in protein, low in carbohydrates, and moderate in fat. The premise of the diet is the protein-fat-carbohydrate mixture that is geared to stimulate fat burning and, like the Atkins Diet, put the body into a safe state of ketosis. The Scarsdale Diet is 43% protein, 22.5% fat, and 34.5% carbohydrates. Unlike the Atkins Diet, however, Tarnower calls for dieters to eat less fat so that as the body "demands more fat, it pulls it out of the fat storage areas." This low-carbohydrate, high-protein diet proclaims that chemical reactions in the food combinations offered in the daily menus lead to weight loss. Tarnower claims the diet plan would help people to lose an incredible one pound per day.

Unlike most other diets, the Scarsdale Diet does not stress the need for daily exercise. Tarnower says that if the diet is followed accordingly, you should shed unwanted pounds without ever exercising.

How it Works

It is simple to follow as it has a meal plan mapped out. A seven- to 14-day plan clearly outlines the types of foods to be consumed at three meals each day. When following the Scarsdale Diet, a strict meal plan must be adhered to. There is no room for improvisation or modification of the menus if you want to lose the amount of weight promised by the plan. Snacking is not allowed, and herbal appetite suppressants and artificial sweeteners are encouraged to speed weight loss. Meals consist of fruit, vegetables, and lean sources of protein in unlimited amounts. There is no calorie counting, but meals are limited to breakfast, lunch, and dinner.

This diet plan also demands that you drink lots of water. The water is used to flush out your system and causes the weight to drop off faster. Alcohol should be restricted to one and one-half ounce a day.

Seven-Day Meal Plan

Breakfast – The same every day: ½ grapefruit, one slice of toast, coffee or tea.

Monday – Lunch: lean cold cuts, tomato slices, coffee or tea. Dinner: broiled fish, salad, one slice of toast, grapefruit, coffee or tea.

Tuesday – Lunch: fruit salad (any kind and as much as you like) and coffee. Dinner: steak or hamburger (without bread), tomatoes, lettuce, celery, olives, Brussels sprouts or cucumbers, coffee or tea.

Wednesday – Lunch: tuna fish or salmon salad with lemon and vinegar, grapefruit, coffee or tea. Dinner: two lamb or pork chops, celery, cucumbers, tomatoes, coffee or tea.

Thursday – Lunch: two eggs, cottage cheese, cooked cabbage, one slice of toast, coffee or tea. Dinner: cold chicken, raw or cooked spinach, coffee or tea.

Friday – Lunch: assorted cheese slices, raw or cooked spinach, one slice of toast, coffee or tea. Dinner: broiled fish, salad (as many vegetables as desired), one slice of toast, coffee or tea.

Saturday – Lunch: fruit salad, coffee or tea. Dinner: cold chicken without skin, tomatoes, grapefruit, coffee or tea.

Sunday – Lunch: hot or cold chicken, tomatoes, carrots, cooked cabbage, broccoli or cauliflower, grapefruit, coffee or tea. Dinner: plenty of steak, celery, cucumbers or Brussels sprouts, tomatoes, coffee or tea.

Advantages

- With the Scarsdale Diet you don't have to count calories or grams of fat, and there is no limit on portion sizes.
- Weight loss often occurs rapidly, and you won't have to worry about hunger.

Disadvantages

- The Scarsdale Diet doesn't advocate exercise for weight loss and recommends no strenuous exercise for those over 40, unless exercise has already been an integral part of the day. The limited caloric intake provides inadequate fuel for anyone hoping to even walk vigorously for 30 minutes a day.

- It's a strict meal plan, with restricted food choices.

- Herbal appetite suppressants can be dangerous for people with heart disease or high blood pressure and have been linked to death when used in large amounts or in conjunction with other stimulants such as caffeine.

- The daily average of 1,000 calories barely provides the body, with enough energy for an average active person.

- One of the major drawbacks of this diet involves estimating how many carbohydrates to eat in a day. This is quite hard, if not impossible to do.

- Any diet that limits carbohydrates causes the body to rely on fat or muscle for energy. When our body breaks down stored fat to supply energy, byproducts called ketones are formed. Ketones suppress appetite, but they also cause fatigue, nausea, and a potentially dangerous fluid loss. In severs cases it can cause unconsciousness and, even lead to a coma. Anyone with diabetes, heart, or kidney problems should NOT follow a diet that promotes the formation of ketones, including the Atkins plan.

- People with diabetes taking insulin are at risk of becoming hypoglycemic if they do not eat appropriate carbohydrates.

- People who exercise regularly may experience low energy levels and muscle fatigue from low carbohydrate intake.

- Eating unlimited amounts of fat, especially saturated fat found in meat products, can lead to increased risk of heart disease in the long term.

- The Scarsdale Diet doesn't conform to the American Heart Association's dietary guidelines for a healthy heart.

- Adherence to the Scarsdale Diet can result in vitamin and mineral deficiencies such as vitamin B, calcium, and potassium.

- Restricting carbohydrates means eating a low-fiber diet, which can cause constipation.
- The diet lacks in phytochemicals derived from carbohydrate-rich plant foods, which are important cancer-fighting agents.

Summary

The Scarsdale Diet, like other low-carbohydrate, high-protein plans, eliminates foods that are high in fiber and many nutrients in favor of quick weight loss. The Scarsdale Diet results in weight loss because the daily calorie intake has been decreased dramatically, with the recommended amount being only 1,000 calories per day. Medical experts suggest a gradual loss of one pound per week is a healthy goal, in contrast to the Scarsdale Diet average of one pound per day.

Although the Scarsdale Diet was one of the first low carbohydrate diets, it has lost popularity to other low carbohydrates programs such as the Atkins Diet or the Zone Diet.

49

Shape Up Diet

Overview

The Shape Up Diet is inspired by Dr. Phil McGraw's book *The Ultimate Weight Solution: Seven Keys to Weight Loss Freedom*. It's billed as a tough-love manual that recommends a balanced approach to weight management consisting of high-fiber foods—including complex carbohydrates, whole grains, fruits, and vegetables—balanced with lean protein and healthy fats.

As such, the Dr. Phil's Shape Up Diet is not about counting calories, points, or fat grams but instead it is about feeding your body and mind with the right kinds of foods—the foods that will help you achieve and maintain the weight that's best for you. Dr. Phil believes this is the best approach to providing a base for losing weight and improving your health without being hungry, compromising good nutrition or being unable to sustain your energy levels.

One of the most crucial tenets of the plan is its reliance on a diet of what Dr. Phil calls "High-Response-Cost, High-Yield foods." High-response-cost foods take time to prepare, can't be eaten quickly, are difficult to digest, and are not considered "convenience foods." On the other hand, a low-response-cost, low-yield food takes very little time to prepare and is high in calories. Dr. Phil says to concentrate on high-response-cost foods since they require more work to take in, the body digests them more effectively, and therefore they don't become stored fat.

How it Works

The Shape Up Diet targets healthy thinking as well as healthy eating. To make choosing the correct foods even easier, the Shape Up Diet program is based around pre-planned menus that consist of portions that are just the right size for you. Weight loss aids such as supplements, nutrition bars and shakes are also available.

Dr. Phil coaches that once you unlock what he refers to as "The 7 keys to self-control," you will never revert to overeating.

In his book, Dr. Phil McGraw addresses the seven steps to what he calls the "no diet plan."

1. The Right Thinking – the individual must change how he perceives his weight.
2. Healing Feeling – he must stop emotional eating and quit sabotaging his efforts to lose.
3. No Fail Environment – he must discover what triggers cravings and eliminate easy access to food.
4. Mastery Over Food – he must do away with impulse eating.
5. High Response Cost Nutrition – he should fill his plate with high-fiber, nutritious foods.
6. Intentional Exercise – in order to shape up, the dieter must get exercise.
7. Circle of Support – his chance of success is greater if he surrounds himself with supportive people

Advantages

- The Shape Up Diet promotes weight loss.
- The diet recommends healthy foods for the most part.
- Most of the foods Dr. Phil's diet recommends support a sound behavioral approach to weight management.

Disadvantages

- Dr. Phil's line of dietary supplements, shakes, and nutrition bars are expensive.

Summary

Dr. Phil's Shape Up Diet offers practical weight-loss advice, but it is nothing other than the guidelines that the American Heart Association, American Dietetic Association, American Diabetes Association, and other major health organizations have been advocating. These organizations give diet advice, recipes, motivation tips, and exercise advice.

Nutritionists have problems with the assumption that Dr. Phil makes that everyone who is overweight has emotional problems or is an emotional eater. For some people, excess weight is the result of too little exercise, poor food choices, and other factors that don't necessarily have to do with emotions.

They also question Dr. Phil's claim that Shape Up Diet meal replacement shakes contain "scientifically researched levels of ingredients that can help you change your behavior to take control of your weight." The supplements found in these shakes for all practical purposes are run-of-the-mill powder made from milk, fiber, and vitamins.

50

Slim-Fast Diet

Overview

The Slim-Fast Diet as seen on TV is based on meal replacement products that are formulated to provide balanced nutrition. It's a structured plan that allows people to have three regular meals and snacks. Two of the regular meals, breakfast and lunch, use Slim-Fast meal replacement products. Dinner, referred as the "sensible meal," is made up of regular foods with emphasis on portion control and following standard nutrition guidelines.

The Slim-Fast meal replacements are different flavored smoothies or meal bars and there are the Slim-Fast snack bars. The products are fortified with vitamins and minerals and provide a good source of protein, carbohydrate, fat, and fiber. All can be bought at major supermarkets. The meal replacements and snack bars can be supplemented with fruit and no-calorie drinks.

Ideally, the plan will help people to lose the healthy level of one to two-pounds a week, but heavier people, especially men, may lose more. This diet is commonly recommended for severely overweight people.

How it Works

Slim-Fast offers two diet plans: the Slim-Fast Optima Diet and the newer Slim-Fast Lower Carb Diet.

The Slim-Fast Optima Diet involves eating six times per day, which includes: two Slim-Fast Meal Combinations, one sensible meal, fruits and vegetables, and snacks if your weight is greater than 140 pounds. The Slim-Fast Meal Combination lets you combine your favorite foods along with a full line of Slim-Fast products (smoothies or meal bars) to create a Slim-Fast meal combination for breakfast and/or lunch. The Slim-Fast Meal Combination along with the smoothies and meal bars includes healthy food choices like a half sandwich, yogurt with fruit, or even a grilled chicken Caesar salad with light dressing. For your sensible meal, one-quarter of your plate should be filled with lean protein, one-half of your plate with vegetables, and one-quarter with carbohydrates. You can also eat a salad on the side and fruit for dessert. A salad with fat-free dressing can be eaten too. You should drink plenty of water and other calorie-free drinks and be active for a total of 30 minutes each day.

The Slim-Fast Lower Carb Diet involves eating six times per day, which includes: two Slim-Fast Meal Combinations, one sensible carbohydrate-conscious meal, fruits and vegetables, and snacks if your weight is greater than 140 pounds. The Slim·Fast Meal Combination is a Slim·Fast Meal (smoothies or meal bars) plus other healthy food choices like a half sandwich, yogurt with fruit, or even a grilled chicken Caesar salad with light dressing. For your carbohydrate-conscious meal, fill two-thirds of your plate with a variety of vegetables, plus one-third part lean protein. A salad with fat-free dressing can be eaten too. You should drink plenty of water and other calorie-free drinks and be active for a total of 30 minutes each day.

Advantages

- Slim-Fast gives the dieters a very structured eating pattern. For some, this can make it easier to follow than diets with a wider range of food choice.

- Slim-Fast (like any minimum 1,200 calorie diet plan) can almost guarantee weight loss. Slim-Fast is one of the few diet companies to back up its products with the gold standard in diet research—controlled clinical trials.

- Slim-Fast provides a wealth of information on lifestyle changes, exercise plans, healthy meal and snack ideas, and weight maintenance.

- Their website includes an online support club an "Ask the Dietitian" section for ongoing support.

- They put strong emphasis on a flexible program designed to fit any individual needs, and their smoothies and bars provide a balanced diet for just about anyone.

- Liquid meal replacements are low fat and often fortified with most vitamins and minerals.

- The smoothies and the snacks taste good, so this diet doesn't seem punitive in nature.

- The Slim-Fast Diet is appealing because of its simplicity and convenience. There's minimal meal planning and the meal replacements in a can or in a bar can be carried and consumed almost anywhere without having to deal with the problems in food preparation.

Disadvantages

- The Slim-Fast Diet can also be costly, as you do have to buy its products.

- Some people may not enjoy the smoothies, although there are plenty of flavors, including juice-based smoothies.

- Like all meal-replacement plans, the Slim-Fast Diet doesn't focus on the big issue of being overweight—the need to learn healthier eating habits. So even though Slim-Fast can almost guarantee weight loss, it does little to ensure that the weight stays off by teaching you good long term eating habits.

- People who like to cook and enjoy fresh foods may be turned off by the convenience-style products.

- Slim-Fast's informational brochures do mention physical activity, but they don't emphasize it enough.

- The Slim-Fast Diet may be a useful starting point for some people, but it offers very little education or advice about entering the real world of fast food, restaurants, and family get-togethers.

- The diet does not offer tips for permanently adjusting eating habits without completely abandoning everything familiar.

Summary

The Slim-Fast Diet, as liquid diets go, is one of the more responsible plans and has been medically tested as a means of losing weight. Following the guidelines set out by Slim-Fast will allow you to lead a healthy and balanced lifestyle, and it steers well clear of any crash weight loss techniques that can result in medical complications.

If you follow the plan as suggested, a 1,200 to 1,500 calorie diet should result in a gradual weight loss for most dieters. However, for anyone who is extremely overweight, 1,200 to 1,500 calories may be too low to begin with, and Slim-Fast offers no formula for increasing the calorie level. There are some medically supervised programs, such as Optifast, that offer much lower calorie levels, but because they are medically supervised, the dieter is being regularly monitored for any potential complications.

Nutritionists have mixed feelings about the Slim-Fast Diet. Some think the program is not a good choice for long-term dieting and question whether any liquid diet actually can train people to eat right. Others believe the Slim-Fast Diet can be an acceptable supplement if dieters remember to eat fruits, vegetables, and whole grains as part of their one daily meal. Keep in mind that bars and smoothies can never provide all the benefits of real food—so use caution when thinking long-term.

51

Somersizing Diet

Overview

The Somersizing Diet was developed by TV celebrity Suzanne Somers. The Somersizing Diet is a mixture of several ideas, as it is part food combining and part Atkins-style low-carbohydrate diet. It eliminates several refined foods, including sugar and white flour—what she refers to as "funky foods"—and recommends separating the rest into "Somersized Food Groups" for mixing and matching. Fruits should be eaten alone on an empty stomach, while vegetables should be eaten with fats and proteins, but never eat proteins and fats with carbohydrates. Somers maintains that when proteins, fats, and carbohydrates are eaten together, their enzymes "cancel each other out," creating a halt in the digestion process and causing weight gain. There is no portion control and the diet recommends eating frequent small meals.

The Somersizing Diet closely resembles other high-protein, low-calorie diets like Protein Power, the Atkins Diet, and the Beverly Hills Diet.

How it Works

The main component to Somersizing is eating the right foods in the right order/combination, unlike almost all of the other low-carbohydrate diets. The seven Somersizing steps are:

1. Eliminate funky foods.
2. Eat fruits alone on an empty stomach.
3. Eat proteins and fats with vegetables.
4. Eat carbohydrates with vegetables but no fat.
5. Keep proteins and fats separate from carbohydrates.
6. Wait three hours between meals if switching from a meal of proteins and fats to a carbohydrate meal or vice versa.
7. Eat three meals a day.

These rules are supposed to help the body metabolize what you eat in a more efficient way, thereby helping you lose weight. Somers cautions dieters to never skip meals—this can and will slow down your metabolism.

Funky foods include a number of food items, including all sugars from white and brown to corn syrup, molasses, honey, maple syrup, white flour, white rice, corn, potatoes, sweet potatoes, butternut squash, beets, carrots, avocados, bananas, nuts, olives, liver, coconuts, milk, and soy-based products. And of course caffeine and alcohol are considered funky foods.

Advantages

- The Somersizing Diet emphasizes frequent small meals and incorporates ways to "splurge" and enjoy your favorite foods without losing control completely.
- There is no need to monitor portions, calories or grams of fat.
- Healthful fruits and vegetables are encouraged.
- Reducing intake of sugar and refined foods will help increase the consumption of more healthful nutrients.

Disadvantages

- The Somersizing Diet is a strict meal plan, with restricted food choices.
- Eating unlimited amounts of fat, especially saturated fat found in meat products, can lead to increased risk of heart disease in the long-term.
- Some people may find following the strict food-combining regimen difficult.
- There is no scientific evidence to suggest that food-combining assists weight loss.
- People with diabetes taking insulin are at risk of becoming hypoglycemic if they do not eat appropriate carbohydrates.
- People who exercise regularly may experience low energy levels and muscle fatigue from low carbohydrate intake.

- The Somersizing Diet doesn't conform to the American Heart Association's dietary guidelines for a healthy heart.

- Another potential problem is that, because it is somewhat restrictive in the nature of the carbohydrate foods it allows, the Somersizing Diet may not always be easy to follow, especially when eating away from home.

- If you go back to a higher carbohydrate diet again, the pounds will return.

- Studies show that restrictive diets, which eliminate several foods or food groups, have the worst failure rates over time—a pretty dismal outlook.

- This is a difficult program to follow long-term for those who enjoy eating sweets, breads, fruits or other carbohydrate-containing foods

Summary

The Somersizing Diet should help you lose weight, because it follows a low calorie plan that eliminates junk food. However, there is no clinical evidence to support the idea that food-combining causes weight loss. Second, there is no evidence that when proteins and carbohydrates are eaten together, their enzymes "cancel each other out," thus creating a halt in the digestion process and causing weight gain. The body contains enzymes that are specifically keyed to individual proteins, carbohydrates, and fats. These enzymes do not cancel each other out, as Somers claims, because they remain in different areas of the digestive tract. Furthermore, if digestion did not occur, the resulting lack of protein and carbohydrate absorption would most likely result in weight loss, not the weight gain as Somers predicts. Third, Somers' advice not to drink water with meals because it dilutes the digestive juices and slows digestion is not supported by any scientific evidence. Fourth, Somers' statement—that no reliable long-term studies have shown any negative effects associated with increased fat consumption— is not true.

South Beach Diet

Overview

The South Beach Diet was developed by Dr. Arthur Agatston, a famous cardiologist and author of *The South Beach Diet*. The origins of the South Beach Diet lay with Agatston, whose motivation was to improve the cholesterol and insulin levels of his patients that had heart disease by developing a healthy eating plan. While the South Beach Diet is lumped together with other low-carbohydrate plans, it takes a decidedly different and healthier approach to protein and fat. The South Beach Diet works on the principle that weight gain is caused by a diet high in saturated fats and processed carbohydrates.

Agatston contends that weight loss is just one of the priorities of the diet (the other is healthful levels of cholesterol and other blood fats). The South Beach Diet educates us to rely on a healthy balanced eating regime between "healthy carbohydrates" (such as whole grains, fruit, and vegetables) and unsaturated fats (such as olive oil). By following this way of eating, the plan promises a reduction in LDL (bad) cholesterol and triglyceride levels, along with increases in HDL (good) cholesterol. Unlike the popular Atkins Diet, this diet does not entail drastically cutting back on a particular food group, i.e. carbohydrates. That's why some call it the "updated version of the Atkins Diet." Exercise, although recommended as with most healthy eating plans, is not a necessity. However, it can help to speed up your weight loss.

Omega-3 fatty acids—polyunsaturated fats found in coldwater fish, canola oil, flaxseeds, walnuts, almonds, and macadamia nuts—also count as good fats. There is evidence that omega-3 fatty acids help prevent or treat depression, arthritis, asthma, and colitis and help prevent cardiovascular deaths. With the South Beach Diet you'll eat both monounsaturated fats and omega-3 fatty acids in abundance in all three phases.

Agatston recommends that you avoid eating low-fat prepared foods (e.g., dairy products such as cheese, milk, and yogurt).

Highly processed foods (refined carbohydrates) like bagels, cornflakes, white bread, potatoes, and soft drinks are the bad guys on the South Beach Diet. These foods are digested and absorbed very quickly, causing a surge in blood sugar levels and resulting in the release of a large amount of insulin. This causes blood sugar levels to drop rapidly, leaving you lacking in energy, craving more carbohydrates, and quickly feeling hungry so that you eat again. If this pattern is frequently repeated, you're likely to gain weight as a result of constantly overeating. But on top of this, over time the body becomes resistant to the action of insulin and when this happens, the body becomes more effective at storing fat.

In contrast, carbohydrates with a low glycemic index release sugar into the blood, providing a steady supply of energy and leaving you feeling satisfied for longer. This means you get fewer carbohydrate cravings and don't constantly feel hungry, so are less likely to overeat. Plus there's less chance that your body will become resistant to the effects of insulin, with the result that it continues to burn fat efficiently. Foods with a low GI are therefore recommended if you want to lose weight.

How it Works

The South Beach Diet works in phases. The first phase lasts for two weeks, the second phase lasts until you've reached your target weight, and the third phase lasts for life. Each phase includes specific meal plans and recipes. The diet also encourages three meals a day, as well as regular healthy snacks. Satisfying your hunger is an important part of this plan.

South Beach Diet Phase 1: Rapid Weight Loss Phase

Phase 1 is the strictest part of the South Beach Diet and lasts for two weeks. Many foods are prohibited during this time, and dieters should expect a rapid weight loss. The goal is to eat three balanced meals a day, and to eat enough so that you don't feel hungry all the time. Drinking plenty of water is required. The first phase is aimed at banishing your cravings for sweets and baked goods.

Foods you can eat include tenderloin, sirloin or top round, skinless chicken or turkey breasts, all types of fish and shellfish, boiled ham, Canadian bacon, turkey bacon, whole eggs, low-fat cheeses, peanuts and pistachios, green vegetables, canola and olive oils, and legumes.

Foods to avoid during the first two weeks include beef rib steaks, honey-baked ham, breast of veal, all yogurt, ice cream, milk, including whole, low-fat, soy, and full fat cheeses; beets; carrots; corn; yams; fruits and fruit juices; all alcohol, and all starchy foods, such as bread, cereal, oatmeal, matzo, rice, pasta, potatoes, pastries, baked goods, crackers, etc.

After the initial two weeks are up, you can begin adding the excluded foods back into your diet.

Expected Weight Loss: 8–13 pounds per week.

South Beach Diet Phase 2: Liberal Phase with Reintroduction of Good Carbohydrates into Diet

Phase 2 of the South Beach Diet is similar to the first phase, but you gradually reintroduce some of the banned foods. There is no time scale set for this phase; you should remain on it until you have reached your target weight. If you regain some weight, switch back to Phase 1 until you lose it. The key here is to re-introduce these foods in moderation and to not eat them as often as you were before.

Foods you can eat also include, most fruits, fat-free or 1% milk, other low-fat dairy foods, high-fiber cereal, whole-grain breads, pinto beans, and red wine.

Diet foods you can eat—sparingly—include refined wheat baked goods, potatoes, beets, carrots, bananas, pineapple, watermelon, and honey.

Expected Weight Loss: 1–2 pounds per week.

South Beach Diet Phase 3: Weight Maintenance

Phase 3 of the South Beach Diet is the most liberal phase, where you make the diet a way of life by focusing on foods with a low or medium glycemic index (GI) and limit foods with high GI. The objective of this phase is to maintain your optimum body weight. You can have snacks or eat food with a high GI if you like them; however, you are only allowed to consume these foods moderately. Should your weight begin to climb, you simply repeat the whole process starting from Phase 1 of the South Beach Diet.

Advantages

- The South Beach Diet encourages three balanced meals, plus snacks if necessary, and allows a lot of flexibility in food choices.
- There's a welcome emphasis on whole grains, fruits, and vegetables that is often lacking in many low-carbohydrate diet plans.
- The diet promotes rapid initial weight loss.
- It helps to improve eating habits and stabilize blood sugar levels.
- Studies have shown that the diet can help to reduce cholesterol as well as decrease the risk of cardiovascular problems.

Disadvantages

- The South Beach Diet lacks options for people who don't like or can't eat dairy. Many snacks are dairy-based, yet the diet bans soy in the first two weeks.
- The glycemic index is used to encourage the consumption of certain types of grains, fruits, and vegetables. But major U.S. health associations, such as the American Diabetes Association and the American Dietetic Association, do not endorse using the glycemic index for weight control or in planning menus for people with diabetes. Eliminating some healthy foods just because they have a high glycemic index number doesn't make sense for every person.
- Some people may follow Phase 1 for long periods of time, which can cause deficiencies of several nutrients, including fiber and calcium.
- Much of the initial 8 to 13 pound weight loss in Phase 1 is likely to be water weight loss caused by carbohydrate restriction. Losing this much water can throw your electrolyte balance off.

- Most of the world outside America thrives on complex carbohydrates and these foods do not cause people to become overweight, nor do they warrant a 14-day ban during Phase 1. In this way, Agatston is helping to perpetuate the American fear of carbohydrates.

Summary

Nutritionists consider Phase One too restrictive. The main safety concern is that the initial two-week phase induces ketosis. Risks associated with ketosis include loss of glycogen stores, dehydration, dizziness, heart palpitations, fatigue, lightheadedness, constipation, irritability, and electrolyte imbalance. You should consult your physician before starting the South Beach Diet if you have a history of heart disease, diabetes, or kidney disease, and are significantly overweight. But Phase 2 and the Maintenance Phase promote healthful fats, lean proteins, and complex carbohydrates, albeit a smaller percentage of them.

Nutritionists are generally in favor of diets based on the glycemic index, but while most believe in eating more foods with a low GI value, they don't necessarily think all high-GI foods should be banned. This is because the GI value of a meal changes considerably when foods are eaten together. That said, few experts would argue with a diet that recommends cutting down on processed carbohydrates and swapping foods rich in saturates for those containing monounsaturated fats.

Critics are less happy with the recommended rate of weight loss. General guidelines recommend losing no more than two pounds a week for good health, so experts are concerned that this diet promotes such a large weight loss in the first two weeks. They say this is unhealthy and is simply the result of a severe calorie restriction caused by cutting out all carbohydrates. As for losing weight from your midsection as the diet claims, most nutrition and fitness experts believe it's impossible to lose fat from just one part of your body.

In general, the South Beach Diet only requires serious willpower for the first two weeks during Phase 1. Once you get past the initial phase, however, there are fewer dietary restrictions than some other diet plans. No major food groups are eliminated, plenty of fruit and vegetables are recommended, and generally the diet follows the basic principles of healthy eating with the result that it should provide plenty of the nutrients you need to stay healthy. In the long term, this is one of the better diets—especially if you avoid Phase 1 and start on Phase 2.

53

Special K Diet

Overview

The "Special K Diet" is nothing more than a marketing campaign by Kellogg's food-company in order to extol the healthful virtues of its fortified bran cereal.

How it Works

The diet works as follows: Eat one cup of Kellogg's Special K, Kellogg's Special K Red Berries, or Kellogg's Smart Start with two-thirds of a cup of skim milk and fruit for breakfast, and again for either lunch or dinner for a total of two weeks. Snack on fruit or vegetables throughout the day. By following a regimen of decreased calorie consumption, any food-specific diet will work.

Advantages

- Eating Special K cereal with skim milk is a great way to add calcium to your diet, and studies have shown that adequate calcium intake (from food, not necessarily from supplements) helps people lose weight.
- Eating breakfast on a regular basis also aids weight loss.

Disadvantages

- Some people may become bored by the repetition in the Special K Diet.
- Special K is one of the healthier cereals out there and an excellent choice as a breakfast meal, but focusing on it in such a narrow manner is not sustainable in the long term.
- In addition, Special K isn't a great source of fiber, nor is it a whole-grain cereal. You'll need to eat plenty of fruits and veg-

etables throughout the day, as well as one or two whole-grain choices at your non-cereal meal (such as brown rice pilaf or a slice of whole-grain bread) to meet your fiber needs.

Summary

This is a kick-start plan, designed to boost weight loss and help you adopt healthier eating habits, such as eating breakfast every morning and choosing more fruits and vegetables. Kellogg's recommends working with a registered dietitian to develop a healthy, long-term weight loss plan.

54

Step Diet

Overview

The Step Diet, authored by James O. Hill, Ph.D., promotes a balanced diet that stresses daily exercise (walking) and cutting back on food portions to lose weight and keep it off for life. Hill is a co-founder of the National Weight Control Registry and an advisor on obesity to the National Institutes of Health. Hill argues that most diets ultimately fail because they provide only a temporary solution, not a permanent way to change lifestyle habits.

Hill believes the key to losing weight under this plan is to make some simple changes that you can live with, set reasonable goals for yourself, and exercise more. Hard workouts aren't necessary; in fact, to keep weight off, you need to take at least 10,000 steps a day. (The book even comes with a pedometer to count your steps.) That's about five miles, but includes the steps you take during the regular course of your day as well as additional exercise. (A few equivalencies: 1 minute of cycling = 150 steps; 1 minute of swimming = 96 steps; 1 minute of yoga = 50 steps.)

The thinking behind the Step Diet is based on the core concept of energy balance: if you want to lose weight, the calories you consume cannot exceed the calories you burn through metabolism and exercise. The Step Diet does not focus on counting calories or eating particular foods. Instead the Step Diet shows you a simple way to reduce your energy intake to lose weight and, most importantly, it shows you a simple way to compensate for the drop in your metabolism that occurs when you lose weight. This plan is about making changes to your lifestyle that you can live with for good.

How it Works

The principles of the Step Diet to losing weight is to eat smaller food portions, gradually increasing the number of steps you walk throughout the day to increase your energy expenditure. No food is off-limits. In combination with exercise, reducing your food intake by one-quarter you will lose weight at a safe rate of one to two pounds per week. Once you have lost the weight, the Step Diet shows you how to manage and maintain the weight loss by helping you determine how many daily steps you need to take to balance the food you eat.

The Step Diet shows you how to increase the number of steps you walk to continue to burn the energy necessary to maintain your weight loss for life. The secret of the Step Diet is that it doesn't focus on food or physical activity as most diets do, but rather on energy balance—the balance between food and activity. All of this can be achieved with two simple tools, a bathroom scale and the Step Counter. If you can maintain energy balance at your desired weight, you will succeed at long-term weight maintenance.

The Step Diet makes this easy by focusing on these steps:

- BodySteps – The energy burned through your body's resting metabolism, converted into steps.
- LifeSteps – The energy burned through physical activity, or steps measured by the Step Counter.
- MegaSteps – The total energy your body burns. (BodySteps + LifeSteps = MegaSteps)

Step Diet Stages of Weight Loss (Time to complete)

Stage 1: Prepare for permanent weight management (Seven days)

Stage 2: Stop gaining weight (Two weeks)

Stage 3: Set your personal weight-management goals (One day)

Stage 4: Make small changes to lose weight (Twelve weeks)

Stage 5: Find your personal energy balance point (Four weeks)

Stage 6: Plan for lifelong success!

Advantages

- The Step Diet is easy to follow.
- The diet helps promote weight loss.

- The diet by promoting exercise strengthens bones, lowers blood pressure, fights cancer, improves immune function as well as fights heart disease.

Disadvantages

- The Step Diet doesn't change your eating habits, which is the number one secret of permanent weight loss.

Summary

All in all, the Step Diet represents an easy to follow plan, a life-long weight management program that can help those struggling with an overweight or obesity problem to overcome. The diet doesn't make any promises, but it does provide answers grounded in research and a straightforward plan for incorporating more exercise into your daily life.

55

Subway Diet

Overview

Subway is a popular fast food brand with outlets worldwide. Subway is known for its 6- or 12-inch "subs" (long rolls or sandwiches) with a large choice of fillings and their own baked breads. The association of Subway with other diet plans came about due to the fantastic weight loss success of Jared Fogle. Jared effectively lived on a diet of low-calorie Subway subs and achieved outstanding weight loss (he began with a weight over of 400 pounds and ended at around 190 pounds). It is worth noting that this diet was combined with a lot of aerobic activity (he was known to have walked a lot). That being said, after receiving plenty of media attention many others have followed in Jared's footsteps and begun what is known as the Subway Diet.

The Subway sandwich chain doesn't endorse the weight loss plan popularized by Jared, but they have capitalized on his success. Jared has been all over TV and billboards advocating the subway diet. Instead of promoting a specific plan, the Subway website provides basic healthy weight loss suggestions such as loading up on as many veggies as possible, eating a healthy breakfast, eating slowly and enjoying your food, choosing calorie-free beverages, and regular exercise.

How it Works

People on the Subway Diet start the day off with coffee. When lunchtime comes around you have a six-inch low-fat sub with baked potato chips. For dinner, you eat a 12-inch veggie sub. The subs are ordered without mayonasise and without cheese. You can choose among the seven subs with six grams fat or less: Veggie Delite, Roast Beef, Turkey Breast, and Oven Roasted Chicken Breast. This is the diet, and it's easy to see that it's not hard to follow.

Advantages

- If fast food is your a way of life, then Subway is definitely a healthy choice.
- Subway is healthy food, and it is prepared for you (which takes a lot of the guesswork out of meal planning and low fat cooking).

Disadvantages

- A Subway-only diet over a long period of time could result in vitamin and mineral deficiencies—cheating you of essential calcium, zinc, and vitamin D.
- In addition, Subway foods can be high in sodium if you add pickles, olives, or salt.
- Eating sandwiches for two meals a day, day in and day out, may get boring.

Summary

The truth is Subway offers a good selection of low-calorie subs, which are excellent for midday lunches or occasional snacks, especially if you're trying to lose weight. The problem with the Subway Diet is that it is far too narrow in its focus and not sustainable in the long-term. It does not teach balanced nutrition that can be adapted to a normal diet once the weight loss goal is reached. As a result, you'll have to supplement these subs with other foods, like fruit and vegetables, or your health may suffer—never mind your weight. Although, to be fair, fast-food addicts and (perhaps) college students could do a lot worse eating at other fast food restaurants where there is no regard for the calories per serving.

56

Sugar Busters Diet

Overview

The Sugar Busters Diet is based on the premise that sugar can cause digestive problems, as well as being a major factor in weight gain. The authors say too much sugar causes the body to overproduce insulin, a hormone that regulates blood sugar levels and fat storage. Excess insulin production leads to increased amounts of body fat and weight, and stimulates the liver to make cholesterol.

The theory behind this diet is that by balancing the insulin-glucagon relationship in the body you'll lose body fat regardless of your calorie intake. Insulin is a hormone produced by the body to lower blood sugar when it gets too high, and glucagon is a hormone produced by the body to raise blood sugar when it goes too low.

The diet just doesn't stop at the sugar jar but also recommends avoiding high-glycemic foods (those that have the greatest effect on blood sugar levels) such as potatoes, corn, white flour, pasta, white rice, and cake. The Sugar Busters Diet recommends eating low-glycemic carbohydrates such as high-fiber fruits, vegetables, whole grains, and lean meats. The lower a food's glycemic index, the less affect it has on blood sugar levels and the better it is for weight loss, according to the Sugar Busters Diet.

In lieu in cutting back on carbohydrates, the Sugars Busters Diet encourages eating high-protein foods such as meats, nuts, and some vegetables. The high protein foods will prompt the body to use up previously stored fat cells.

The Sugar Busters Diet also recommends food combining. For instance, the authors recommend that you eat fruits by themselves, not in combination with other carbohydrates. This diet plan does not require counting calories, weighing foods, or calculating grams of carbohydrates, but you are expected to balance the portions on your plate.

How it Works

The Sugar Busters Diet is easy to follow and, if you follow their 14-day diet exactly, you should lose weight. The plan is similar to those of many other low-carbohydrate plans: 40% carbohydrates, 30% protein, and 30% fat. The New Sugar Busters book mentions that you can increase carbohydrates to 50% as long as the choices are low-GI foods.

While on this diet, you are allowed to eat red meat, poultry, fish, olive oil, dairy foods, and nuts. There are certain fruits and vegetables you can eat as well. The authors of the diet claim that this diet discourages—and is in fact wary of—saturated fats, not only because they can cause weight gain, but because of the effect they can have upon vital organs, the heart in particular. They also advise that all meat should be lean and should have the fat trimmed off it. The authors recommend cooking with oils that are high in mono- and polyunsaturated fats and low in saturated fats, such as canola. High fiber foods are also encouraged in this diet, although some high fiber foods, such as bananas, are prohibited because they also contain high levels of sugar. As mentioned, you must also eliminate potatoes, corn, white rice, bread from refined flour, beets, carrots and, of course, refined sugar, corn syrup, molasses, honey, and sugared colas. Oats, small amounts of whole-grain bread, and whole-wheat pasta are also permitted. If you choose alcohol, you should drink red wine.

Listed below is a typical meal plan for a Sugar Busters Diet.

Breakfast
- An orange or one-half grapefruit
- Hot oatmeal or whole-grain cereal
- Coffee or tea

Lunch
- Turkey and Swiss cheese on whole-grain bread with mustard and/or mayonnaise, lettuce, and tomato
- Diet drink, tea, or water.

Dinner

- Grilled or baked meat such as pork tenderloin, salmon or other fish, chicken, veal, steak, or lamp chops
- Whole-wheat pasta sprinkled with Romano or Parmesan cheese, and brown rice
- Steamed fresh yellow or spaghetti squash and/or zucchini
- Romaine lettuce salad with fresh snow peas, roasted pine nuts, and a dressing of olive oil, balsamic vinegar, a little chopped garlic, basil, and a dash of Creole mustard
- Water, coffee, tea, diet drinks, and milk are okay to drink during the day. Snacks can include nuts, grapes, two thin slices of cheese, and sugar-free ice cream or frozen yogurt

Advantages

- The Sugar Busters Diet gives clear guidelines on which foods to avoid.
- The diet helps to eliminate consumption of refined sugar.
- This diet does not involve calorie counting.
- Because the diet recommends eating low-glycemic carbohydrates such as fruits, vegetables, and whole grains, you'll be taking in lots more vitamins, minerals, and phytochemicals.

Disadvantages

- The Sugar Busters Diet downplays the idea that calorie intake causes weight gain or weight loss.
- There is no scientific justification for the premise that healthy people who eat foods high in sugar will automatically gain weight.
- Lumping foods such as bananas, potatoes, corn, and carrots with the "forbidden" sugars makes no nutritional sense.
- Sugar is not toxic and insulin does not lead to weight gain.
- The diet also eliminates some valuable minerals and nutrients.

- The diet restricts some fruits and vegetables, which are essentially for a healthy diet.
- The authors downplay the importance of physical activity. In fact, activity is all but dismissed as a waste of time in the battle of the bulge, something that research strongly contradicts.
- Dieters with a sweet tooth often sabotage dieting efforts.
- Very little dairy is included in the Sugar Busters Diet plan, so it's likely to be low in calcium and vitamin D.

Summary

Any diet that encourages high-fiber foods such as whole grains, fresh fruits, and vegetables in place of candy and refined flour products is applauded by nutritionists. However, when otherwise-healthy fruits and vegetables like pineapple, raisins, carrots, and bananas are restricted because they make blood sugar levels rise too quickly, you have to wonder about the logic of the diet. Also, the idea that sugar is toxic to the body is complete nonsense; although sugar has no nutritional value and counts as "empty calories," it is in no way toxic.

The most controversial claim of the Sugar Busters Diet is that insulin resistance can be reduced, by eliminating or severely restricting certain foods. Insulin resistance is a condition wherein our bodies have become insensitive to normal levels of circulating insulin in the bloodstream. Normally, a small amount of insulin will control blood sugar levels, but with insulin resistance, larger and larger amounts of insulin are pumped into the blood in an effort to lower blood sugar. Medical experts assert that the diet does not cause insulin resistance but that it is rather caused by obesity.

The general consensus among dieticians is to tightly control the number of carbohydrate grams you eat each day rather than worry about the source of those carbohydrates. Total carbohydrate intake is what's important for controlling sugar and insulin levels.

Overall, the Sugars Busters Diet is low in fiber and high in fat and cholesterol and is not recommended as a long-term eating plan.

T-Factor Diet

Overview

The T-Factor Diet, developed by Dr. Martin Katahn, claims dieters can lose weight safely and quickly without cutting back or counting calories by eating a higher proportion of carbohydrates to fats. Katahn's premise is based on the "thermogenesis" and "thermic effect of foods" or the T-Factor, the way the body generates heat by burning carbohydrates, fats, and proteins at different rates. In simple terms, studies on thermogenesis suggest that fat in the diet turns into body fat more easily than carbohydrates in the diet. Thus, the higher the proportion of carbohydrates to fats in the foods you eat, the lower the chances of gaining excess fat. In simple terms: you can eat as much as you want as long as you cut down on fat.

Katahn maintains that in order to maximize the body's T-Factor level the dieter should focus on the source of calories eaten rather than the total number of calories consumed. This simply means the dieter must eat low-fat foods instead of fatty foods. Total calories consumed—whether from fat, carbohydrate, protein, or alcohol—still count.

How it Works

Katahn recommends an intake of 20 to 40 grams of fat a day for women and 30 to 60 grams a day for men for weight loss, which is about 15 to 20% of our calories from fat. Dieters wishing to lose weight faster should cut their fat intake to 20 grams for women and 30 grams for men.

Listed below are some of the foods that might be found in a typical T-Factor Diet.

Breakfast
- Banana or fresh fruit
- Dry cereal
- Skim milk

- Coffee or tea

Lunch

- Cottage cheese
- Raw vegetables
- Whole-wheat crackers
- Fresh fruit

Dinner

- Baked chicken
- Brown or wild rice
- Salad with fat-free dressing
- Fruit

Snacks

- Nonfat yogurt
- Fresh fruit
- Low-fat crackers

Katahn recommends whole body exercises such as walking, swimming, or biking rather than start-stop exercises such as tennis, or aerobics. He believes start-stop activities burn more carbohydrates than fat, while continual whole-body movements burn fat more than carbohydrates.

Advantages

- The T-Factor Diet promotes rapid initial weight loss.
- The diet stresses the importance of exercise in losing or maintaining weight.

Disadvantages

- Critics argue it is too difficult to follow the T-Factor Diet since it recommends that only 15 to 20% of daily calories come from fat. Americans currently eat closer to 40% of their calories as fat and are having trouble getting down even to the recommended 30% level.

Summary

Nutritionists give the T-Factor diet high marks for being well-balanced, with plenty of fruits, vegetables, and whole grains. However like other low-fat, high-fiber diets, like the Dr. Dean Ornish, Dr. John McDougall, and Nathan Pritikin diets, the T-Factor diet has been criticized by medical experts for being too difficult to follow because it is too low in fat. To put this into perspective, consider that a one-ounce slice of cheddar cheese or a three-ounce serving of salmon provide about nine grams of fat; one table-spoon of oil, butter, or margarine, 12 grams of fat; or three ounces regular ground beef has 18 grams of fat. It's easy to see how quickly fat adds up and how difficult it would be for the dieter not to exceed the daily intake of calories from fat. Thus, it's doubtful that many dieters who follow Katahn's advice will be able to lose weight "painlessly and easily," as he promises.

58

Total Wellbeing Diet

Overview

The Commonwealth Scientific and Industrial Research Organization (CISRO) developed a high-protein, low-fat diet that recommends moderate consumption of nutritious whole grains and other low glycemic index (GI) carbohydrate foods. Known as the "Total Wellbeing Diet," its goal is to provide sound nutrition for life, and not simply be a short-term diet for weight loss.

How it Works

When the desired weight has been achieved, and food intake must be slightly increased to maintain the new (reduced) weight, the Total Wellbeing Diet recommends that this extra food should come mostly from whole-wheat breads and cereals. The recommendation is also made that some of the additional food should come in the form of low-fat milk or other dairy products and nutritious snack foods (e.g., nuts, fruit bars, and low-fat pizzas).

Advantages

- The Total Wellbeing Diet also emphasizes the need to be active, and provides useful tips on how you can achieve adequate levels of activity.
- It may be a healthier and effective alternative to the more orthodox high-carbohydrate, low-fat diets for losing excess body fat.

Disadvantages

- Although the CSIRO diet claims to be the Total Wellbeing Diet, it does not address all the nutritional problems faced by many Australians. It is also important to adhere to those aspects of the

Dietary Guidelines for Australians not mentioned in the Total
Wellbeing Diet.

Summary

In summary, although the Total Wellbeing Diet is new, and hasn't yet been
subjected to long-term testing for efficacy and safety with some nutritionists believing it to be better than other high-protein diets. However, as noted
with other high-protein diet plans, such diets are not considered suitable
by most orthodox nutritionists. Most nutritionists emphasize the importance of lowering intake of fat (particularly saturated fat), and increasing
consumption of vegetables, fruits, and cereal foods such as bread, rice, and
pasta—preferably whole-grain.

59

Vegetarian Diet

Overview

A Vegetarian Diet includes only foods from plants: fruits, vegetables, legumes (dried beans and peas), grains, seeds, and nuts. However, the eating patterns of vegetarians may vary considerably. The lacto-vegetarian diet includes plant foods plus cheese and other dairy products. The lacto-vegetarian excludes eggs as well as meat, fish, and fowl. The lacto-ovo-vegetarian (or ovo-lacto-vegetarian) diet also includes milk, cheese, yogurt, and eggs, but excludes meat, fish, and fowl. Those who eat eggs but no dairy, by contrast, are called ovo-vegetarians. Semi-vegetarians don't eat red meat but include chicken and fish with plant foods, dairy products, and eggs. And those who choose to eat no animal products at all are called vegetarians. This form of vegetarianism is often referred to as a vegan (pronounced vee-gun or vee-jan) diet.

Some macrobiotic diets fall into the vegan category. Macrobiotic diets restrict not only animal products but also refined and processed foods, foods with preservatives, and foods that contain caffeine or other stimulants.

Common reasons for choosing a vegetarian diet include health considerations, concern for the environment, and animal welfare factors. Vegetarians also cite economic reasons, ethical considerations, world hunger issues, and religious beliefs as their reasons for following their chosen eating pattern.

How it Works

In planning vegetarian diets of any type, one should choose a wide variety of foods to ensure the adequate intake of certain nutrients, which may be limited unless care is taken to choose reliable sources. These nutrients include proteins, calories, vitamins D and B12, and minerals such as calcium, iron, and zinc in the correct amounts for growth and for good health. These elements can be found in any vegetarian diet, but it is necessary to understand how they fit together to plan a healthy diet.

Vegetarians can meet their need for protein by choosing a variety of protein-containing foods. Plant proteins alone can provide enough of the essential and non-essential amino acids, as long as sources of dietary protein are varied and caloric intake is high enough to meet energy needs. Whole grains, legumes, vegetables, seeds, and nuts all contain both essential and non-essential amino acids. Textured vegetable proteins and meat analogues (usually made from soybeans and fortified with amino acids) are good protein sources.

Eating enough whole grains and legumes throughout the day will give the body the calories it needs for energy.

Vitamin B12 comes naturally only from animal sources. Vegetarians should have a reliable source of vitamin B12, because it is needed for normal red blood cell formation and normal nerve function.

Iron deficiency is a common problem in vegetarian and non-vegetarian diets. Women need high quantities of iron in their daily diet to prevent anemia. Good sources of iron include tofu, beans, lentils, split peas, and other legumes, figs and dried fruit, nuts, fortified cereals and breads, enriched pasta, and dark green leafy vegetables. Iron is better absorbed when these foods are consumed with vitamin C-rich foods (e.g., citrus fruits, tomatoes, and broccoli). Try to avoid drinking black tea with meals, as it inhibits iron absorption.

Vitamin D deficiencies may be a problem for people who are not exposed to direct sunlight. Vitamin D is added to fortified soy and rice beverages, fluid milk products, and margarines, but is not found in yogurt or cheeses. Check the label before making purchases.

The best sources of riboflavin are liver, milk products and red meats. When these foods are restricted or avoided, riboflavin must come from other sources, such as green leafy vegetables and fortified or enriched grains.

Whole-grain breads and cereals as well as brown rice contain phytates, a compound that interferes with the absorption of zinc. As a result, vegetarians generally require more zinc. Legumes, beans, lentils, peas, tofu, cashews, almonds, and fortified vegetarian meats are good sources of zinc.

Iodine is needed for normal functioning of the thyroid gland and associated hormones. Iodized salt is the most common source of iodine in the Western diet. Iodine is found in seawater, so any type of seafood is a rich source of this element, particularly seaweed. Vegetarians or people who do not eat seafood can get iodine from seaweed or iodized salt.

Advantages

- A Vegetarian Diet offers a number of advantages, including lower levels of saturated fat, cholesterol, and animal protein and higher levels of carbohydrates, fiber, magnesium, boron, folate, antioxidants, vitamins such as C and E, carotenoids, and phytochemicals.

- Many studies have shown that vegetarians seem to have a lower risk of obesity, coronary heart disease (which causes heart attack), high blood pressure, and some forms of cancer.

- Vegetarian diets tend to be lower in sodium and higher in fiber than the typical American diet.

- Vegetarians often have weights that are closer to desirable weights than do non-vegetarians

- Vegetarians may be at lower risk for non-insulin-dependent diabetes because they are leaner than non-vegetarians.

- Vegetarians' high intake of complex carbohydrates, which are often relatively high in fiber content, improves carbohydrate metabolism and may lower basal blood glucose levels.

Disadvantages

- The Vegetarian Diet might be considered by some to be monotonous and devoid of taste.

- Some vegetarians may have intakes of vitamin B12, vitamin D, calcium, zinc, and occasionally riboflavin that are lower than recommended.

- Vegetarians may have a greater risk of iron deficiency than non-vegetarians.

Summary

A balanced Vegetarian Diet has been shown to have some very real health benefits. Studies continuously show vegetarians have lower incidences of heart disease, diabetes, high blood pressure, and certain forms of cancer than those whose diet is high in protein. More and more evidence is emerging in favor of the health benefits of a cereal- and grain-rich diet.

People following a typical Vegetarian Diet will loose weight faster than their meat-eating counterparts. This can be attributed to the fact that most vegetarians' diets are comprised mainly of complex carbohydrates. Complex carbohydrates are starchy, fiber-rich foods, and are naturally low in fat.

60

Very Low-Calorie Diet

Overview

A Very Low-Calorie Diet (VLCD) is a short-term weight loss diet for obese people. VLCDs are commercially prepared formulas of 800 calories or less that replace all usual food intake. VLCDs are not the same as over-the-counter meal replacements, which are meant to be substituted for one or two meals a day. VLCDs, when used under proper medical supervision, effectively produce significant short-term weight loss in moderately to severely obese patients.

VLCDs are generally safe when used under proper medical supervision in patients with a body mass index greater than 30. VLCDs are not recommended for pregnant women or breastfeeding women. VLCDs are not appropriate for children or adolescents, except in specialized treatment programs.

How it Works

As indicated, a VLCD is designed only for obese individuals under medical supervision. Under these conditions, it typically produces significant short-term weight loss amounting to three to five pounds per week, or about 44 pounds over 12 weeks. This can improve obesity-related conditions, including diabetes, high blood pressure, and high cholesterol. If combined with behavioral therapy and exercise, such a diet may also retard weight regain.

Advantages

- A VLCD can lead to weight loss for severely- to moderately-obese patients.
- Weight loss can improve obesity-related medical conditions, including diabetes, high blood pressure, and high cholesterol.

Disadvantages

- In the early stages of a VLCD (up to 16 weeks), dieters may experience a few minor side effects such as fatigue, constipation, nausea, and diarrhea, but these side effects usually improve or disappear entirely.

- There are other more serious side effects with this sort of rapid weight loss regimen, including the development of gallstones.

Summary

Anyone suffering from moderate to severe obesity is at an increased risk of developing obesity-related medical conditions. Although VLCDs are efficient for short-term weight loss, they are no more effective than other dietary treatments in the long-term maintenance of reduced weight. Therefore, obese patients should be encouraged to commit to a long-term treatment program that includes behavioral therapy and exercise. Behavioral therapy helps you to recognize what causes you to over-eat so that you can consciously change those behaviors.

61

Volumetrics Diet

Overview

The key to weight management with the Volumetrics Diet lies in the food choices that help you feel full with fewer calories. For more than 20 years, Barbara Rolls, Ph.D. has researched appetite and appetite control. The culmination of her research studies were published in a book, co-authored by Robert A. Barnett, *The Volumetrics Weight-Control Plan*. Rolls believes the absence of satiety, or the sensation of fullness, is one reason why most diets don't work very well or for very long. "The biggest mistake dieters make is that they eat less of everything, and then they feel hungry," says Rolls. Volumetrics is based on the concept of "energy density," which means how concentrated the calories are in a portion of food. High energy density foods provide a large number of calories in a small serving, while low energy density foods provide a small number of calories in a large serving.

Rolls contends that people need to eat more low-energy-dense (few calories per ounce) and a high-volume foods, such as fruits and vegetables, so they get that satisfying amount of food and enough calories. This view is echoed in the 2005 Dietary Guidelines for Americans. The secret ingredients that make foods less energy dense are water and fiber, which explains why most vegetables and fruits are among the lowest-energy foods. The higher the water content and/or the higher the fiber content, the lower the energy density of the food and the more volume the food has, which affects how full you feel. Keep fiber intake high, drink a lot of water, and eat a lot of foods high in water content and low in energy density, and you will lose weight. At the other end of the spectrum are the low-volume, energy-dense foods (which means they have a lot of calories per gram) such as chocolate chip cookies, ice cream, and nuts.

The principle behind the Volumetrics Diet is simple: Eat more foods that have low-caloric density and you'll be able to eat more food, satisfy your hunger, and still cut back on calories. According to Rolls' research, we all tend to eat the same average weight in food every day, no matter how many calories the food contains. With Volumetrics we eat the same volume of food but lower the number of calories by eating foods that are higher in fiber and water.

How it Works

There are no menus to follow and no mandates as to how or when certain foods should be eaten. Instead, Volumetrics contains extensive charts of the energy density (E.D.) and caloric content of any food group. One set of charts is broken down by the USDA Food Guide Pyramid food group and the other set provides listings for beverages, mixed dishes, fast foods, and desserts. The charts are arranged from lowest to highest energy density, making it easy to make good low-calorie, low-density choices. A low E.D. means you can eat more of the food; a high E.D. means you should restrict your intake. Although the charts are extensive, the E.D. of any food can be calculated by dividing the number of calories per serving by the weight in grams per serving.

To use the Volumetrics Diet for weight control, Rolls recommends making up a large portion of the diet with foods that have fewer calories in a serving than their weight in grams, resulting in an energy densities below 1, which includes most fruits and vegetables, and low-fat diary products. Other good foods with calories equal to or slightly greater than their weight, or an energy density between 1 and 2 are beans, fish, chicken without the skin, potatoes, pasta, rice, and low-fat salad dressings. Foods that have two or more times as many calories as their weight are ice cream, beef, French fries, cheese, pretzels, full-fat salad dressings, chips, cookies, bacon, and oils. These foods need to eaten sparingly.

Overall, the diet provides about 20 to 30% of calories from fat, 55% from carbohydrate, and 15% from protein. It also includes 20 to 30 grams of fiber and lots of water—9 cups a day for women and 12 cups a day for men.

Advantages

- Volumetrics helps you understand and overcome overeating without deprivation.

- There's a welcome emphasis on whole grains, fruits, and vegetables that is lacking in many diet plans.
- The diet is not as restrictive as some other diets.
- This is not a weight loss diet, rather a health plan that will assist your body to reach and maintain its optimal weight.
- The diet helps you lose weight while feeling full and satisfied.
- The diet is based on the science of how much people eat, and why.
- The diet is easy to understand and implement.
- You don't have to eat special foods with this diet.

Disadvantages

- The grocery bill for a Volumetrics Diet may be higher. On a per-calorie basis, fruits, vegetables, fish, lean protein, and low-fat diary products are more expensive sources of pure calories.
- People looking for a quick fix won't find it with this diet.
- Energy density is not listed on food labels.

Summary

Overall, the Volumetrics Diet receives good ratings from nutritionists because it encourages eating more fruits, vegetables, whole grains, legumes, and beans, and eating less high-fat, low-nutrient junk foods. If you have trouble controlling your weight and tend to overeat, the Volumetrics weight control plan will help you eat less without deprivation. If you are true to the Volumetrics' formula for eating, you should feel satisfied and still lose weight.

Warrior Diet

Overview

Ori Hofmekler, founder and editor-in-chief of the health and fitness magazine *Mind and Muscle Power*, created the Warrior Diet. Hofmekler explains his Warrior Diet in terms of following the instinctive eating cycle of an ancient warrior, which was cycling between under-eating during the day and overeating at night.

Hofmekler believes most diets disregard human survival instincts and therefore make no biological sense. It's these survival instincts that regulate the ability to control healthy eating habits giving us a real sense of hunger. Any diet that saturates your body with too many meals will keep you from having this primal sense of hunger. Without it, you lose your ability to manage instinctual eating habits. Without primal hunger, people don't have any real sense of what to eat and how much, and when to stop eating.

Under-eating during the day forces the body to redesign itself for a better metabolic efficiency thus activating a full spectrum of essential hormonal and enzymatic activities. Under this condition, the body reaches peak potential to assimilate nutrients while acquiring a real sense of hunger for food to survive. Overeating at night from all food groups will give you a feeling of full satisfaction with a great sense of freedom. Historically, night was the time to eat and a way of tightening social bonds, and a time to relax from the stress of daily activities.

Hofmekler stresses strength over size, leanness over unnecessary bulk. He says that in order to achieve a fully conditioned body you must have strong joints as well as a strong back. He compares the dieter's body to that of a Roman solider. Hofmekler believes that anyone who follows his diet plan correctly will become more alert, sharper, and more energetic. They will become a warrior and possess the warrior instinct.

How it Works

The Warrior Diet is based on a daily feeding cycle of "under-eating" during an eight-hour day to burn fat, and "overeating" at night. The Under-eating Phase during the day would maximize the sympathetic nervous system (SNS) that regulates the "fight or flight" mechanism that enables you to react under stress. The SNS keeps you alert, focused, and agile. The Over-eating Phase at night would maximize the parasympathetic nervous system (PNS) recuperation effect on the body, and thereby promote calm, relaxation, digestion, and the utilization of nutrients for repair and growth.

The Under-eating Phase

The Under-eating Phase is built on the principle of controlled fasting. It lasts for 16-18 hours after your last meal, including the time you are asleep. During this phase, you can consume fresh, raw fruits and vegetables, and some protein, or in extreme cases not eat anything but only drink water, coffee, or tea. The extreme methods usually don't appeal to most people. Hofmekler recommends the best way of going through the Under-eating Phase is to follow a controlled fast since it's easier to follow and it accelerates detoxification and overall well-being. The goals of the Under-eating phase are:

- Burn fat and repair tissues
- Detoxify and cleanse the body
- Manipulate hormones to reach maximum metabolic efficiency

With a controlled fast, insulin drops and the hormone glucagon increases to ensure a steady supply of energy to the body. When this occurs most of the body's energy is derived from glycogen reserves and fat stores. Also, the drop in insulin allows the growth hormone (GH) to peak, which helps the body to rejuvenate, repair tissues and burn fat. A natural elevation of GH on a daily basis should help slow the aging process.

The Overeating Phase

The Overeating Phase involves following your instincts, which will give you a sense of freedom and real satisfaction. Eat as much as you want from all the food groups (protein, fats, and carbohydrates), as long as you follow the Warrior Diet rules of eating:

- Start with leafy green vegetables
- Continue with protein, cooked vegetables, and fat such as olive oil, almonds, avocado, and butter
- Finish with carbohydrates
- Stop eating when you feel much more thirsty than hungry

The goals of Overeating phase are:

- Accelerate your anabolism (repairing tissues and building muscles)
- Boost your metabolism
- Replenish your glycogen reserves
- Nourish your body and mind for pleasure and full satisfaction (compensation)
- Retrain to eat instinctively

Advantages

- The Warrior Diet, being rich in fruits and vegetables, is rich in antioxidants, which have been shown to lower the risk of cancer and heart disease.
- There isn't much meal planning involved since everything you eat is raw fresh fruit and vegetables.

Disadvantages

- There is no real assurance that you will lose weight following this diet plan.
- The constant fasting and eating can be disruptive to your digestive track.

- The Warrior Diet can be addicting because there's a certain feeling that comes from going without food or having an enema—almost like the high other people get from nicotine or alcohol.

- It's not recommended for people with diabetes, low blood sugar, or eating disorders.

- The Warrior Diet can be especially risky for people who are involved in sports and physical activities that require ample food.

Summary

The general consensus is that the Warrior Diet is probably effective in temporary and quick weight loss, but is not effective for long-term weight loss. The obvious criticism of the Warrior Diet is the fasting during the day and binging at night. People who have special dietary needs, including diabetics, should definitely consult a doctor before starting the Warrior Diet.

Nutritionists argue that Hofmekler's theory about eating as our ancestors purportedly being a healthy way to eat lacks solid scientific support. They point out no research has been done that supports his claim.

63

Weigh Down Diet

Overview

The Weigh Down Diet was created by Gwen Shamblin, a dietitian who struggled with her own weight. The basic premise of the diet is that God can take away the desire to overeat. Shamblin believes that overeating is a problem of the soul, and those who focus on God and prayer can and will lose weight.

How it Works

The diet program does not discuss what specific foods should be eaten, nor does it encourage dieters to cut out bad foods. Instead, dieters focus on when they are physically hungry as opposed to when they are spiritually hungry. The program uses fasting as a way of gaining more control over eating problems.

Advantages

- The Weigh Down Diet helps you lose weight while leading a spiritual life.
- There isn't much meal planning involved since you can eat practically anything you want.

Disadvantages

- Medical experts question the Weight Down Diet's use of fasting and lack of insight into its related risks. Fasting is sometimes an early sign of anorexia or bulimia.

Summary

The main philosophy behind the program is good, but the diet offers no upfront nutritional information or regimentation.

64

Weight Watchers Diet

Overview

Probably the most recognized of the organized weight loss programs, Weight Watchers, founded by Dr. Jean Nidetch, has been around since a humble beginning in Queens, New York, in 1963. Though Weight Watchers has changed a lot over the years, it has remained steadfast in its goal of offering weight loss guidance in a group support environment while emphasizing a balanced diet and encouraging exercise. At local group meetings, Weight Watchers' members get motivation, mutual support and encouragement in handling the challenges encountered in the process of changing behavior.

Weight Watchers has produced its own line of cuisine, which may be purchased independently at most major grocery chains. There is a one-time registration fee and a weekly fee.

How it Works

The Weight Watchers program is based on calorie reduction using the Weight Watchers Points system. Foods are assigned a certain number of points according to their calorie count, the number of fat grams they contain, and their fiber content. The higher the fat grams the more points assigned to that food. The higher the fiber grams the fewer the points assigned to that food. Dieters are allotted a certain number of points, referred to as the Daily Point Range, that is determined by their body weight and the number of pounds they want to lose. Dieters must record all foods eaten and their point value every day to make sure they're staying within their assigned points. Stay within the Daily Points Range and you'll lose weight. The number of points each dieter is alloted daily ranges from 18 to 35 points, which is based on their body weight, and how much weight they are trying to lose. For example, a 5'6" woman who weights 180 pounds would be allotted between 22 and 27 points each day.

Weight Watchers is extremely flexible about the foods you can eat; in fact, you can literally eat anything and lose weight, so long as you keep track of your points and don't exceed your Daily Point Range. For example, one cup of grapes counts as one point, one scoop of ice cream as four points, and one slice of pizza as nine points. The more points you use on a single item, the fewer foods you'll be able to eat during the day. Although the choices are left to the dieter, Weight Watchers leaders and materials offer considerable guidance for choosing a healthy and nutritious diet.

The key is properly calculating the points of various foods, which can be done by using the provided Weight Watchers food lists and points calculators. Portion size is determined by either weighing food to stay within the required parameters, or by becoming familiar with various equivalents. For example, a serving of meat should be no larger than the palm of your hand, and a serving of rice should be about the size of a tennis ball. Here are some examples:

1 cup broccoli = 0 points

1 cup of grapes = 1 points

1/2 cantaloupe = 2 points

1 small bean burrito = 5 points

1 cup spaghetti with 1/2 cup marinara sauce = 6 points

1 6-ounce steak = 8 points

1 3-ounce grilled chicken breast = 3 points

1/4 cup regular creamy salad dressing = 8 points

1 slice bread = 2 points

1 ounce chocolate = 4 points

1 scoop vanilla ice cream = 4 points

1 slice of pizza = 9 points

Members can earn extra bonus points with exercise. Based on a formula that factors in body weight, time, and intensity, all types of physical activity can be assigned a points value. For example, if a woman walks or cycles at moderate intensity for 30 minutes, she would earn two points for her workout.

Weight Watchers menu plans typically include lots of fruits, vegetables, whole grains, and low-fat dairy products. Though Weight Watchers sells entrees, desserts, and snacks in supermarkets, dieters are not required to buy them to participate in the diet plan. Once you've lost the weight and have begun maintenance, your points are adjusted upward as necessary and you continue to attend the same group meetings for support.

Weight Watchers recommends that dieters do some sort of activity at least 30 minutes each day and is especially enthusiastic about the benefits of walking.

Group support has been the cornerstone of the Weight Watchers program since its inception. Most dieters follow the Weight Watchers program by attending weekly meetings. The meetings include a private confidential weigh-in, and they give dieters a chance to exchange suggestions, ideas, and strategies, and to receive advice from the class organizer. Those who don't have a local Weight Watchers group or don't have time to attend one don't have to go it alone. They can receive online support at the Weight Watchers website: www.weightwatchers.com.

The Core Plan

Recently Weight Watchers unveiled the first major change to its diet plan by adding a new weight-loss program that focuses on nutritious food that fills stomachs without packing on calories. The Core Plan, as it is called, consists of a list of approved items from every food group that can be eaten with almost no regard to portion size. The new program resembles certain other diet programs, notably the Volumetrics weight plan, in that it focuses on high-volume foods with a low energy density. The Core Plan will focus on broth-based soups, as well as leaner meats, fresh produce, whole grains and nonfat dairy products. As with Weight Watchers' current system, it includes menu suggestions at popular restaurants.

Advantages

- Dieters participating in the Weight Watchers program generally lose as much weight as those who used their own do-it-yourself approach.

- The group support the Weight Watchers program provides is one of its strongest features.

- The Weight Watchers Points system is a good program, which balances proper nutrition, counseling and exercise. Dieters are never left hungry or feeling lethargic—in fact, dieters often report they are eating more on Weight Watchers Points program than normally. The food consumed is just more nutritious.

- The Winning Points Plan does an effective job of teaching portion control and educates the dieter on the nutritional value of foods.

- The advantage of the Weight Watchers plan is that it not only helps people limit caloric intake, but it also allows for optimal nutrient intake.

- A stellar medical advisory board, with some real heavy hitters from the weight-loss and exercise arenas, keeps the company on the cutting edge of weight-loss research.

- Weight Watchers groups are found virtually everywhere, including many work locations and online.

Disadvantages

- The Weight Watchers Points system can be abused. Someone could potentially spend a whole day's points on ice cream or junk food.

- Calorie counting does raise our awareness of the relative caloric value of foods. However, calorie content is only one standard of measurement. A candy bar may contain the same calories/points as a large sandwich, but it's not as healthy or nutritious.

- It's difficult to continue counting calories for the rest of your life. There comes a time when you must be able to survive without counting points.

- Many dieters obtain great benefits from meeting other dieters and talking through their problems. But some find it less beneficial.

Much depends on the personality and experience of the Weight Watchers meeting organizer. If you are especially sensitive about your weight, it might be best to leave the class before the discussion period, or skip classes altogether and consider joining the Weight Watchers at-home program instead.

Summary

Overall, the Weight Watchers Diet generally receives good ratings from nutritionists because its emphasis is on moderate fat and balanced nutrients. Typically, people who follow the Weight Watchers Points program over a period of time will lose weight. While, on average, participants lost only small amounts of weight while enrolled in the structured Weight Watchers Points program, some participants can lose considerably more weight, with the maximum amount of weight loss reaching about 50 pounds. Many believe the structured program has its advantages over trying to lose the weight on your own.

65

What Color is Your Diet

Overview

David Heber, M.D., Ph.D., founding director of the UCLA Center for Human Nutrition, created the What Color Is Your Diet. This diet is more for cancer prevention and is not specifically a weight-loss diet. Heber recommends a diet with fruits and vegetables across the spectrum of color to get the full range of benefits. Fruits and vegetables have unique properties that provide combinations of substances with unique effects on human biology.

Government health experts say that people should get a minimum of five servings a day of fresh produce. However, Heber believes simply eating five servings a day of fruits and vegetables will not guarantee that you are eating enough of the different substances needed to stimulate the metabolic pathways of genes in the different organs where fruits and vegetables have their beneficial effects. As a result, Herber created a color guide system for fruits and vegetables to make it easier to consume the proper amount and types of vitamins needed in our diets. Heber says that simply counting servings may not be adequate if you are missing out on one or more major color category since not all members of the fruit and vegetable group are alike.

How it Works

Herber's "Color Code" system is as follows:

Red Group

These foods contain the carotenoid lycopene, which helps rid the body of free radicals that damage genes. Lycopene seems to protect against prostate cancer as well as heart and lung disease. Processed juices contain a lot of the beneficial ingredients. One glass of tomato juice gives you 50% of the recommended lycopene for one day. Examples: tomatoes, V8 Juice, watermelons, and pink grapefruit.

Orange Group

These foods contain beta-carotene, which protects against cancer. Examples: carrots, mangos, apricots, cantaloupes, pumpkin, acorn squash, winter squash, and sweet potatoes.

Yellow/Green Group

These foods are rich sources of the carotenoids lutein and zeaxanthin, which are believed to reduce the risk of cataracts and age-related macular degeneration. Examples: spinach greens, collard greens, mustard greens, turnip greens, yellow corn, green peas, honeydew melon, and avocados.

Orange/Yellow Group

These foods contain vitamin C, which protects cells, and beta-cryptoxanthin, which helps cells in the body communicate and may help prevent heart disease. Examples: pineapple, orange juice, oranges, tangerines, peaches, papayas, and nectarines.

Red/Purple Group

These foods are loaded with powerful antioxidants called anthocyanins, believed to protect against heart disease by preventing blood clots. They may also delay the aging of cells in the body. There is some evidence they may help delay the onset of Alzheimer's disease. Examples: purple grapes, red wine, blueberries, cranberries, blackberries, strawberries, red apples, beets, eggplant, grape juice, and prunes.

Green Group

These foods contain the chemicals sulforaphane and isocyanate, and they also contain indoles, all of which stimulate liver genes to make compounds that break down cancer-causing chemicals. Examples: broccoli, Brussels sprouts, cabbage, bok choi, and kale.

White/Green Group

These foods contain flavonoids, which protect cell membranes. Examples: leeks, scallions, onions, garlic, celery, pears, white whine, endive, and chives.

Advantages

- Nearly all fruits and vegetables are low-fat and contain fiber and natural chemicals known as phytonutrients that can help protect against heart disease, cancer, age-related cognitive decline, cataracts, and macular degeneration.

Disadvantages

- Eating five to nine portions of vegetables and fruits a day—about a pound a day—may be hard for some people to stomach.

Summary

Eating too much of anything—even colorful vegetables—is not healthy eating. But most Americans won't have trouble with eating too much of these healthy foods. A wide range of nutritionists endorse Heber's recommendations that people should eat a lot of different vegetables and fruits.

66

Zone Diet

Overview

The Zone Diet created by Barry Sears, Ph.D. is basically a high-protein diet plan. The Zone Diet's strategy calls for a return to the diets of our ancestors where meat, fruits, and vegetables are the main dietary items. Sears maintains a high-protein low-carbohydrate diet decreases hunger and consequently weight. Unlike the Atkins Diet, the Zone Diet allows greater carbohydrate intake. Sears recommends consuming 40% of your daily caloric intake in the form of carbohydrate and 30% as protein, with fat making up the other 30%. Sears even pits his plan against the Atkins Diet, insisting that his does better at alleviating hunger and generating mental and physical energy. Like the Atkins Diet, the protein intake recommended is higher than that advised by any major health organization.

Sears claims that we as a society are overweight due to a high intake of carbohydrates, especially high-glycemic-index carbohydrates, and that this style of eating causes an over-production of insulin resulting in weight gain. In addition to causing weight gain, excess insulin can be linked to other aspects of ill health, such as heart disease, cancer, and arthritis. Sears asserts that by using the Zone Diet you can control your insulin production by eating the proper ratio of low-glycemic carbohydrates, dietary fat, and protein. Maintaining your insulin level within a therapeutic "Zone" makes it possible for you to burn excess body fat (and keep it off permanently), and enjoy increased energy and improved mental focus, while alleviating the symptoms of multiple sclerosis and AIDS.

How it Works

The Zone Diet does not actually prohibit you from any particular food group as long as you balance carbohydrates with protein in the Zone 40:30:30 ratio. To help with this, "Zone Food Blocks" have been developed, where each block contains a standardized amount of carbohydrate, protein, or fat. To lose weight, a certain number of blocks are allocated for each meal and snack. The number of Zone Food Blocks you should have each day is calculated according to your weight, height, and waist and hip circumferences. Generally, the bigger you are, the more blocks you are allowed. The diet generally ends up providing about 800 to 1,200 calories a day, which Sears calls a "Zone-friendly" diet plan.

In simple terms, the Zone Diet involves cutting out most carbohydrates such as breakfast cereals, rice, potatoes, pasta, noodles, bread, bagels, croissants, muffins, crisps, pastries, pies, chocolate, sweets, sugar, and preserves, as these have the greatest effect on blood sugar levels and therefore insulin levels. Most fruits and vegetables, however, are allowed. Low-fat protein-rich foods such as skinless chicken, turkey, and fish should be eaten with every meal with the portions being relatively small. Finally, most of the fat should consist of heart-healthy monounsaturated fat (such as from olive oil, almonds, and avocados). Unlike high-protein diets (that induce ketosis) or high-carbohydrate diets (that elevate insulin levels), the insulin control component of the Zone dietary program is based on balance and moderation at each meal. The other component of the Zone dietary program is supplementation with high-dose fish oil.

The Basic Zone Diet Rules

- Make sure every meal and snack has the right combination of low-fat protein, the appropriate type of carbohydrate (preferably fruits and vegetables), and a small amount of "good" fat (like nuts or olive oil).

- Always eat a Zone meal within one hour after waking.

- Eat five times per day: three Zone meals and two Zone snacks.

- Never let more than five hours go by without a Zone meal or snack (whether or not you are hungry). In fact, the best time to eat is when you aren't hungry because that means your blood sugar levels are stable. Afternoon and late evening snacks are important to keep you in the Zone throughout the day.

- Drink at least eight eight-ounce glasses of water every day.

Advantages

- The Zone Diet encourages you to cut out a lot of the "junk"—low-nutrient carbohydrates in your diet such as crisps, cakes, biscuits, and chocolate.

- Sears claims a person in the Zone will experience permanent body-fat loss, optimal health, greater athletic performance, and improved mental productivity.

- The Zone Diet generally has fewer dietary restrictions than many other low-carbohydrate plans and recommends eating more fruit and vegetables.

- Eating fewer fatty foods—and swapping foods that are high in saturated fats for those containing monounsaturated fats—is sensible, heart-healthy advice, too.

- Advocates of the Zone Diet claim you can lose at least five pounds in the first two weeks, followed by one to 1.5 pounds every week after that.

- Specific meal plans are available to guide you into the Zone.

Disadvantages

- The Zone Diet is very low in carbohydrates, which can quickly sap your energy levels.

- It recommends eliminating some very nutritious foods, which are not only a good source of carbohydrate but are also packed with fiber and important vitamins and minerals. For example, whole-grain cereals are packed with fiber, B vitamins, and iron, while cheese is an excellent source of calcium and zinc.

- It can be expensive if you decide to purchase pre-packaged Zone products.

- The health risks, like heart disease and cancer, are similar to the Atkins Diet, though not as much since the Zone Diet allows for more healthy carbohydrates, such as vegetables and fruits.

- You may drop pounds quickly, but you may regain them just as fast once you go off the diet.

- You can't feed your family the same thing, because they will have different calculations.

- Considered too complicated because you have to weigh every single ingredient before preparing it.

- Although counting calories is not a part of the diet plan, if the diet is strictly followed, the daily calorie intake could be too low to provide all the nutrients necessary for good health.

Summary

It's great that the Zone Diet promotes monounsaturated fats like olive oil, olives, and peanuts, as well as the omega-3 fatty acids found in fish oils. However, nutritionists believe a diet of 30% protein is higher than what most health organizations recommend and 40% carbohydrates are slightly lower than advisable. Both the American Dietetic Association and the American Heart Association disapprove strongly of the Zone Diet primarily due to its high protein content, so it is not recommended as the lifelong diet. They assert that the Zone Diet has not been proven effective in the long term for weight loss. They believe that the Zone Diet is hazardous as it restricts the intake of essential vitamins and minerals present in certain foods.

At the heart of the Zone Diet is the claim that eating too many carbohydrates can develop excess insulin resulting in ill health and obesity. Nutritionists argue that excess insulin, a condition known as insulin resistance, is not a consequence of eating too many carbohydrates and they say medical research has not linked insulin levels to weight gain in healthy people.

SECTION II

Diets for Medical Conditions

67

Acid Reflux Diet

Gastroesophageal reflux disease, commonly referred to as GERD, or acid reflux, is a condition in which your esophagus becomes irritated or inflamed when the stomach regurgitates an acidic liquid into the esophagus. The esophagus, or food pipe, is the tube stretching from your throat to your stomach. Your esophagus lies just behind the heart, so the term "heartburn" was coined to describe the sensation of acid burning the esophagus.

Normally, a ring of muscle at the bottom of your esophagus, called the lower esophageal sphincter, prevents reflux (or backing up) of acid. This sphincter relaxes during swallowing to allow food to pass. It then tightens to prevent flow in the opposite direction. With GERD, however, the sphincter relaxes between swallows, allowing stomach contents to well up and irritate the lining of the esophagus. When stomach acid comes in contact with the walls of the esophagus, an uncomfortable pain or burning sensation behind the sternum can result, sometimes radiating toward the mouth. GERD affects nearly one third of the adult population of the United States at least once a month to some degree. Almost 10% of adults experience GERD weekly or daily. Not just adults are affected; even infants and children can have GERD.

One of the simplest treatments for GERD is a change in your diet. Certain foods are known to reduce the pressure in the lower esophageal sphincter and thereby promote acid reflux. Foods that should be avoided include chocolate, peppermint, fatty foods, alcohol, and caffeinated drinks. In addition, people who experience acid reflux may find that other foods aggravate their symptoms. Examples are spicy or acid-containing foods like citrus juices, carbonated beverages (with and without caffeine), and tomato-based products.

There are some easy lifestyle changes related to eating habits that may help reduce the symptoms of acid reflux. Acid reflux is worse following meals. Therefore, eat small frequent meals instead of three big meals a day, and avoid late evening snacks before going to bed. The smaller and earlier evening meals may reduce the amount of reflux for two reasons. First, the smaller meal results in lesser distention of the stomach. Second, by bedtime, a smaller and earlier meal is more likely to have emptied from the stomach than is a larger one. As a result, acid reflux is less likely to occur when we lie down.

In addition, you may be able to reduce the frequency and volume of reflux by taking the following preventative steps:

- Eat slowly and chew food well.

- Drink liquids one hour before or after meals instead of with meals. If you must drink during a meal, sip only small amounts as you eat.

- Reduce your weight if you are overweight since obesity leads to increased reflux.

- Include enough fiber in your diet to avoid constipation, which can lead to an increase in intra-abdominal pressure.

- Avoid chewing gum immediately following meals. The air that you swallow while chewing gum may lead to belching and reflux.

- Stop using tobacco in all forms. Nicotine weakens the lower esophageal muscle.

Acne Diet

Acne develops when the pores in the skin become blocked with dead skin; then fatty materials accumulate within the blocked pore. The pore then becomes infected with bacteria, resulting in inflammation—the pimple.

Scientists have not found a connection between specific foods and acne. The common train of thought "chocolate causes acne" is a myth. There is no scientific link between sugary and greasy foods and pimples; however, it is very important to maintain a healthy diet. The Journal of the American Medical Association recognized that, "Diet plays no role in acne treatment in most patients...even large amounts of certain foods have not clinically exacerbated acne."

There are several nutrients found in foods that promote an overall healthy body. According to the American Academy of Dermatology, "A healthy diet is important for improving raw materials for healthy skin." Vitamin A, a fat-soluble vitamin, helps maintain the integrity of skin and mucous membrane that function as a barrier to bacteria and viruses. The Vitamin A produced by plants, known as beta-carotene, is usually found in yellow/orange fruits and dark green vegetables. Keep in mind that high doses of Vitamin A can be toxic, so control your consumption.

Arthritis Diet

Nearly one in six Americans, or 43 million suffer from arthritis, making it one of the most common diseases in the United States. There are two basic types of arthritis: osteoarthritis and rheumatoid arthritis. Osteoarthritis, the most common form of the disease, is a degenerative condition (a breakdown of cartilage in the joint) that causes stiffness and pain in the joints, and is usually the result of aging. Osteoarthritis is a much less common problem in underdeveloped countries where people work hard throughout life. Rheumatoid arthritis is a chronic inflammatory condition, which causes joints to swell and become painful. The exact cause of rheumatoid arthritis is not known, although one reason for the prevalence of rheumatoid arthritis may be a high-fat, high-cholesterol diet. Indeed, inflammatory arthritis is much more common in countries where rich foods are eaten, like the United States, Canada, Western Europe, Australia, and New Zealand. (In a few people, some plant proteins, such as the gluten of wheat, may also be a contributory cause.)

Although there is no overwhelming scientific evidence confirming the benefits of modified diets for people with arthritis, healthcare providers have recommended a balanced diet, which includes a variety of foods from the four major food groups essential to your well-being. The four food groups are: 1) vegetables and fruits, 2) bread and cereals, 3) milk and dairy products, and 4) lean meats, poultry, and fish.

Try to restrict the amount of fat, salt, and sugar you eat, and eat more fruit, vegetables, breads and cereals. Adequate calcium for people of all ages is important to help protect against osteoporosis, which causes many fractures in older women. Low-fat milk and dairy products are preferable to full-fat types and are widely available.

One of the most important things you can do is to avoid foods high in saturated fats. Studies have shown that an overall healthy diet, with only small quantities of saturated fats (but with higher levels of polyunsaturated fats) brought about improvement in many arthritis patients.

One of the most exciting recent discoveries is that omega-3 fatty acids in the diet help some people with arthritis. These essential fatty acids are found naturally in oily fish, especially mackerel, sardines, pilchards, and salmon. The fish oil seems to work by reducing the number of inflammatory "messenger" molecules made by the body's immune system.

If you think a particular food may aggravate your arthritis, you might try avoiding a specific food or group of foods such as milk, meat, or processed foods. If that helps, those foods can then be gradually reintroduced one at a time to determine what food provoked the symptoms.

People with arthritis often have vitamin and mineral deficiencies, but these deficiencies are thought to be a result of the disease rather than its cause. The most commonly observed vitamin and mineral deficiencies in people suffering with arthritis are folic acid, vitamin C, vitamin D, vitamin B6, vitamin B12, vitamin E, folic acid, calcium, magnesium, zinc, and selenium. Although food is always the preferred source for vitamins and minerals, it may be essential to supplement your diet with vitamins and minerals. Studies involving vitamin and mineral supplements have shown conflicting results with few hard conclusions. Still, there is some evidence that certain supplements may work directly on the inflammation that causes painful joints.

In addition to the usual reasons for watching your diet, medical experts believe obesity may worsen arthritis symptoms. Being overweight does affect people with arthritis. Joints affected by arthritis are already under strain. If you are overweight or obese, the extra load on your joints may be exacerbating your symptoms, especially if your affected joints include those of the hip, knee or spine. There is also a clear link between being overweight and an increased risk of developing osteoarthritis.

70

Attention Deficit Disorder Diet

Attention deficit disorder (ADD) is the most common behavioral problem in children and teenagers. ADD is characterized by an inability to focus or concentrate for extended periods of time. ADHD (Attention Deficit Hyperactivity Disorder), is marked by hyperactive or inappropriate behavior. The condition is 10 times more common in boys than girls. The disorder shouldn't be confused with the normal boisterous behavior of a child. Almost all children with this disorder improve in later childhood, but some remain socially and educationally underdeveloped. Two thirds of children with ADHD still have some problems in adulthood.

Many health professionals advocate identifying the underlying causes of ADD/ADHD instead of rushing into a course of powerful and potentially harmful drugs for people with ADD/ADHD. By addressing the root causes of ADD/ADHD, you can eliminate—or, at the very least, alleviate—the need to place children on stimulant ADD/ADHD medications. All doctors—across the board—agree that ADD/ADHD medications are not the cure for ADD/ADHD, but simply a means of minimizing the symptoms.

No specific food or diet has been clearly shown to have a significant positive or negative effect on the symptoms of ADD/ADHD. That having been said, it may help to follow a varied and balanced diet and probably eliminate particular additives such as caffeine and refined sugar from the diet.

It has been found that many ADD/ADHD children have a deficiency of essential fatty acids (EFAs). This could be either because they cannot metabolize them properly, because they cannot absorb EFAs normally from the gut, or because their EFA requirements are higher than normal.

EFAs are long-chain polyunsaturated fatty acids derived from linolenic, linoleic, and oleic acids. There are two families of EFAs: omega-3 and omega-6 fatty acids.

Alpha Linolenic Acid (ALA) is the principal omega-3 fatty acid, from which the body makes eicosapentaenoic acid (EPA) and later converts it into docosahexaenoic acid (DHA). DHA is very important for the brain. For the conversion from ALA to DHA the body needs an adequate supply of vitamins C, B6, and B3, and enough zinc and magnesium. Consequently, it is recommended to supplement the diet with a multivitamin containing the vitamin B family, along with essential minerals such as copper, iodine, magnesium, potassium, and zinc. Also, if the diet contains too much omega-6 fats in comparison to ALA (as is usually the case in Western diets), then the conversion is slowed down.

The best source of ALA is flaxseed and flaxseed oil as well as hempseed oil, hempseeds, walnuts, pumpkin seeds, Brazil nuts, sesame seeds, avocados, some dark leafy green vegetables (kale, spinach, purslane, mustard greens, collards, etc.), canola oil (cold-pressed and unrefined), soybean oil, wheat germ oil, salmon, herring, mackerel, sardines, anchovies, and albacore tuna. Mackerel reportedly often has high mercury levels.

Parents should speak to a pediatric dietician before removing an important part of a child's diet, because eliminating certain foods may be harmful.

Regular physical activity has been shown to play an important role in some of the common related conditions (e.g., depression, anxiety) and can improve concentration. Regular exercise may be beneficial to people with ADD/ADHD.

71

Bipolar Diet

Bipolar disorder is a mood disorder characterized by alternating states of depression and mania that follow each other in a repeating cycle. People with bipolar disorder may cycle through these states quickly, or may experience long periods of depression or mania. Because of the highs and the lows—the two poles of mood—the condition is referred to as "bipolar" depression. In between episodes of mood swings, a person may experience normal moods.

The manic phases describe the periods when the person feels overly excited and confident. These feelings can quickly turn to confusion, irritability, anger, and even rage. The depression phases describe the periods when the person feels very sad or depressed. Because the symptoms are similar, sometimes people with bipolar depression are incorrectly diagnosed as having major depression. Often one mood state predominates, while the other occurs only infrequently or briefly. The cause of bipolar disorder is unknown.

In addition to taking your medications every day as prescribed, you can help control mood swings by eating a healthy and balanced diet. A balanced diet includes foods from different food groups, including whole grains, dairy, fruits and vegetables, and protein. Eat a variety of foods within each group (for example, eat different fruits from each fruit group instead of only apples). A varied diet helps you get all the nutrients you need, since no single food provides every nutrient. Eat a little of everything, but nothing in excess. All foods can fit in a healthy diet if you eat everything in moderation. Among other recommendations, it has been suggested a diet free of sugar, alcohol, soda, and caffeine may be best. Alcohol should be avoided, since it may trigger episodes and may interfere with your prescribed medicines.

Some studies have suggested the potential mood-stabilizing benefits of omega-3 fatty acids found primarily in fish oil.

You can also help reduce the minor mood swings and stresses that lead to more severe episodes by making a few simple lifestyle changes such as getting enough exercise and getting enough sleep.

72

Cholesterol Lowering Diet

Although your body makes its own cholesterol, some foods such as sea-food, dairy products, and meats contain cholesterol, too. While some cholesterol is needed for good health, too much cholesterol in your blood can raise your risk of having a heart attack or stroke. The extra cholesterol in your blood may be stored in your arteries (blood vessels) and cause them to narrow, which is referred to as atherosclerosis. Large deposits of cholesterol can completely block an artery so the blood can't flow through. If an artery that supplies blood to your heart becomes blocked, a heart attack can occur. Or if an artery that supplies blood to your brain becomes blocked, a stroke can occur.

Cholesterol travels through the blood in different types of packages, called lipoproteins. High-density lipoproteins (HDL) are good for you because they remove cholesterol from the bloodstream. Low-density lipoproteins (LDL) deliver cholesterol to the body. This is why too much LDL cholesterol is bad for the body, while the HDL form is good. It's the balance between the types of cholesterol that tells you what your cholesterol level means (see the box below). Total cholesterol is the amount of HDL and LDL cholesterol found in the blood.

Total Cholesterol Levels
  Less than 200 is best
  Between 200 to 239 is borderline high
  240 or more means you're at increased risk for heart disease
LDL Cholesterol Levels
  Less than 130 is best
  Between 130 to 159 is borderline high
  160 or more means you're at higher risk for heart disease
HDL Cholesterol Levels
  Less than 40 means you're at higher risk for heart disease
  60 or higher reduces your risk of heart disease

Main Contributors in High Blood Cholesterol Levels

Saturated Fats

While medications are often necessary for individuals at high risk of heart disease, what can play a significant role in reducing high cholesterol levels in the blood is a healthy diet. The most important factor to control is the total saturated fat in the diet. For some people, keeping their total fat intake to 30% of the total calories consumed will lower cholesterol levels in the blood. Others may have to reduce fat to 20% of their total calories.

Saturated fats are found in foods such as fatty cuts of meat, poultry with the skin, whole-milk dairy products, lard, and in some vegetable oils like coconut, palm kernel, and palm oils. Saturated fats raise both the good HDL cholesterol levels and the bad LDL cholesterol levels. Unsaturated fats, monounsaturated and polyunsaturated, are found in plant products. They are sometimes called "good fats" because they can raise HDL and lower LDL if they replace other fats in the diet.

Since many foods high in total fat are also high in saturated fat, eating foods low in total fat will help you eat less saturated fat. When you do eat fat, you should substitute unsaturated monounsaturated and polyunsaturated fat for saturated fat. Examples of foods high in monounsaturated fat are olive and canola oils; those high in polyunsaturated fat include safflower, sunflower, corn, and soybean oils.

Dietary Cholesterol

While reducing the amount of saturated fat in your diet, it is also important that you eat foods low in dietary cholesterol. Dietary cholesterol is found in meat, poultry, seafood, and dairy products. Foods from plants—such as fruits, vegetables, vegetable oils, grains, cereals, nuts, and seeds—don't contain cholesterol. Egg yolks and organ meats are high in cholesterol, and shrimp and crayfish are somewhat high in cholesterol. Chicken, turkey, and fish contain about the same amount of cholesterol as do lean beef, lamb, and pork.

Obesity

Exercise goes hand-in-hand with a healthy diet. Physical exercise can raise HDL cholesterol and may lower LDL cholesterol. Being more active can also help you lose weight, lower your blood pressure, improve the fitness of your heart and blood vessels, and reduce stress.

Diet Guidelines for Lowering High Blood Cholesterol Levels

Red Meat and Poultry

Meat and poultry are important sources of protein and other nutrients in your diet. However, they also contain saturated fat and cholesterol. To lower your blood cholesterol level, eat lean meats and poultry without the skin. Remember, all of these foods contain some saturated fat and cholesterol. Therefore the amount you eat is also important. Organ meats, like liver, sweetbreads, and kidneys are relatively low in fat. However, these meats are high in cholesterol. Egg yolks are also high in cholesterol. Eat no more than three egg yolks a week including those in processed foods and many baked goods. Egg whites contain no cholesterol and can be substituted for whole eggs in recipes.

Fish and Shellfish

Most fish is low in saturated fat and therefore is usually a good substitute for meats and poultry. However, shellfish varies in cholesterol content—some is relatively high and some is low—but all has less fat than meat, poultry, and most fish.

Dairy Products

Although many people believe that meats have the highest cholesterol and saturated fat content, dairy products that contain fat are also high in saturated fat and cholesterol. Try eating low-fat dairy products.

Fats and Oils

Unsaturated oils like canola, safflower, sesame, corn, soy, peanut, and olive oil can reduce bad LDL cholesterol without lowering the good HDL cholesterol. Saturated fats like palm oil, coconut oil, lard, and shortening can raise LDL cholesterol levels, as does hydrogenated fats. By using unsaturated oils instead of these other fats, you can fight cholesterol without changing the way you cook.

Fruits and Vegetables

Fruits and vegetables contain no cholesterol and are very low in fat and low in calories (except for avocados and olives, which are high in fat and calories). By eating fruits as a snack or dessert and vegetables as snacks and side dishes, you can increase your intake of vitamins, minerals, and fiber and lower your intake of saturated fat and dietary cholesterol.

Breads, Cereals, Pasta, Rice, and Dried Peas and Beans

Breads, cereals, pasta, rice, and dried peas and beans are all high in complex carbohydrates and low in saturated fat. By substituting more foods from this group for high-saturated fat foods, you will decrease your saturated fat, dietary cholesterol, and calorie intake.

Breads and most rolls are also low in fat (for more fiber, choose the whole-grain types). However, many other types of commercially baked goods, such as croissants, biscuits, doughnuts, muffins, and butter rolls, are made with large amounts of saturated fats.

Sweets and Snacks

Sweets and snacks often are high in saturated fat, cholesterol, and calories. Examples of these foods are commercial cakes, pies, cookies, cheese crackers, and some types of chips.

73

Gluten-Free Diet

A gluten-free diet is essential for people who have been diagnosed by a physician with coeliac disease or dermatitis herpetiformis (a gluten induced skin sensitivity). Some people may choose to follow a gluten-free diet for other reasons, although these two diseases are the only ones where a gluten-free diet is considered medically imperative. Gluten is a mixture of proteins found in wheat, rye, barley, triticale, and oats.

The symptoms of coeliac disease are similar to those of other disorders, but may include:

- Anemia
- Digestive upsets, such as flatulence and bloating
- Diarrhea or constipation
- Nausea
- Vomiting
- Abdominal pains and cramps
- Weight loss
- Fatigue and generalized malaise.

A gluten-free diet means avoiding all foods that contain wheat, rye, barley, triticale, and oats—in other words, most grain, pasta, cereal, and many processed foods. Despite these restrictions, people with celiac disease can eat a well-balanced diet with a variety of foods, including bread and pasta. For example, instead of wheat flour, people can use potato, rice, soy, or bean flour. Or, they can buy gluten-free bread, pasta, and other products from special food companies. Plain meat, fish, rice, fruits, and vegetables do not contain gluten, so people with celiac disease can eat as much of these foods as they like.

The gluten-free diet can be complicated; and it requires a completely new approach to eating that affects a person's entire life. People with celiac disease have to be extremely careful about what they buy for lunch at school or work, eat at cocktail parties, or grab from the refrigerator for a midnight snack. Eating out can be a challenge as the person with celiac disease learns to scrutinize the menu for foods with gluten and question the waiter or chef about possible hidden sources of gluten. However, with practice, screening for gluten becomes second nature and people learn to recognize which foods are safe and which are off limits.

74

Gout Diet

Gout is a form of arthritis that's characterized by sudden, severe attacks of pain, redness, tenderness, and swelling in some joints. Gout strikes when uric acid builds up in the body to such an extent that the kidneys are unable to flush it out. (Uric acid is a substance that normally forms when the body breaks down waste products called purines, which are found naturally in your body as well as in certain foods.) The uric acid crystallizes and then collects around the joints, causing inflammation. Typically, the first area hit is the big toe, to which crystals are drawn by gravity. Gout can be inherited or happen as a complication of some other condition. Insulin resistance may also play a role in the development of gout. Gout can affect anyone of any age, but typically it affects men over the age of 40 and women after menopause.

Treatment of gout used to include severe dietary restrictions. But medications to treat gout have reduced the need for such restrictions. Still, some dietary modifications may help reduce the severity of gout attacks. They may also be useful for people who have problems with gout medications.

A low-purine diet is often prescribed for individuals with gout. Best case: the less purine in your diet, the fewer gout attacks you are likely to suffer. Worst case: the less purine in your diet, the fewer anti-gout drugs you'll need.

Foods to restrict (very high in purines):

- hearts
- herring
- mussels
- yeast
- smelt
- sardines
- sweetbreads

Foods to limit (high in purines)

- anchovies
- grouse
- mutton
- veal
- bacon
- liver
- salmon
- turkey
- kidney
- partridge
- trout
- goose
- haddock
- pheasant
- scallops

Foods to eat occasionally (moderately high in purines, but may not raise your risk of gout):

- asparagus, cauliflower, mushrooms, peas, spinach
- whole-grain breads and cereals
- chicken, duck, ham, turkey
- kidney and lima beans

Foods that are safe to eat (low in purines):

- green vegetables, tomatoes
- fruits and fruit juices
- breads and cereals that are not whole-grain
- butter, buttermilk, cheese, eggs
- chocolate and cocoa
- coffee, tea, carbonated beverages
- peanut butter, nuts

Dairy products that may lower your risk of gout:

- low-fat or skim milk
- low-fat yogurt

Additional dietary considerations include the following:

- Avoid alcohol, or drink in moderation. Alcohol can raise uric acid levels and provoke an episode of gout.
- Drinking 10 to 12 eight-ounce glasses of non-alcoholic fluids every day is recommended, especially for people with kidney stones, to help flush uric acid crystals from the body.
- Maintain a healthy weight, since excessive weight puts more stress on your joints and increases the risk of gout.
- Lose weight if you're overweight, but avoid fasting or rapid-weight-loss diets since they can increase uric acid levels in the blood. Also, avoid low-carbohydrate diets that are high in protein and fat, which can exacerbate gout.

High Blood Pressure Diet

Few people doubt the importance of sodium in ones diet. However, too much sodium (e.g., salt) causes more fluid to be contained in the blood vessels. This increase in the volume of blood within the confines of the circulatory system contributes to a rise in blood pressure. In addition, sodium causes arterioles to constrict more thus increasing blood pressure. High blood pressure can in turn increase the likelihood of heart or kidney disease and stroke.

The amount of sodium needed in a day depends on the individual. A daily sodium intake of between 1,100 and 3,300 milligrams is considered safe and adequate for most individuals. This is equal to the amount of sodium in approximately one-half to one-and-one-half teaspoons of table salt. Many Americans, however, consume two to five teaspoons of salt per day, which can add up to 12,000 milligrams.

The major sources of sodium in our diets are processed foods like frozen dinners, boxed noodle and rice dishes, canned soups, and canned vegetables. Another major source is the salt we add to food during cooking or at meals. Sodium also comes from a variety of other sources. Baking soda, some seasonings, antacids, and condiments can contain large amounts of sodium. Some prescription and over-the-counter drugs also contain sodium. Reading food and medication labels prior to purchase will help you make low sodium choices.

Reducing the Amount of Sodium in Your Diet

Sodium is found naturally (in low amounts) in fresh foods like meats, nuts, grains, fruits, vegetables, and dairy products. These sources of sodium should prove quite sufficient for good health. Fresh fruits and vegetables contain very little natural sodium and can be eaten often.

To minimize the sodium you eat, reduce your intake of processed foods such as soups, ready-to-eat cereals, celery salt, garlic salt, catsup, mustard, sauces, baking powder, baking soda, potato chips, corn chips, tortilla chips, saccharin-flavored soda, and club soda. Sodium is also hidden as a part of other chemical additives, such as sodium nitrite, sodium benzoate saccharin, and monosodium glutamate. Even some drugs have large amounts of sodium in them. Always read the labels on over-the-counter drugs. When in doubt, ask a pharmacist, or your healthcare provider, if the drug is one you can use safely.

Many people add too much salt to their diet purely out of habit. This only encourages a salty-taste. Learn to use spices and herbs that do not contain salt to enhance the flavor of your food. Lemon, lime juice, or vinegar can help brighten up the taste of foods too. When people begin to lower the salt in their diet, their taste begins to change. After a while, food begins to taste better without salt than it did with it.

76

Irritable Bowl Syndrome Diet

Irritable bowel syndrome (IBS) is a disorder that interferes with the normal functions of the large intestine (colon). It is characterized by a group of symptoms: crampy abdominal pain, bloating, gas, constipation, and diarrhea. One in five Americans has IBS, making it one of the most common disorders diagnosed by doctors. It occurs more often in women than in men, usually begins around age 20.

Fortunately, unlike more serious intestinal diseases such as ulcerative colitis and Crohn's disease, IBS doesn't cause inflammation or changes in bowel tissue or increase your risk of colorectal cancer. In many cases, you can control IBS by managing your diet, lifestyle, and stress.

Traditionally any food high in fat, insoluble fiber, caffeine, coffee, and/or alcohol may in fact bring about the symptoms. Some people experience a worsening of their symptoms after they eat certain foods such as dairy products. It is unclear why these foods cause IBS but eliminating certain foods from the diet can do wonders to improve symptoms. Keeping a food and symptom diary or following an allergy avoidance diet may help identify which foods may be problematic.

Sugar maldigestion is another possible dietary cause of IBS. Sugars are normally broken down by specific enzymes in the intestines and then absorbed. Some people, however, don't produce some of these enzymes, so the sugars don't get broken down properly. Consequently, bacteria eat these undigested sugars in the large intestine producing large amounts of gas.

Lactose intolerance, the most common form of sugar maldigestion, occurs in people who can't digest the lactose sugar found in milk. See Lactose Intolerant Diet for more information. Another form of sugar maldigestion is called sorbitol intolerance, which involves the sugar sorbitol. Sorbitol is found in high amounts in certain fruits and juices such as peaches, pears, plums, and apple juice. It is also added to many dietetic products such as sugarless chewing gum, diet soft drinks, and dietetic jams. It's estimated that as much as 43% of Caucasians and 55% of non-Caucasians are sorbitol intolerant. Reducing the intake of these foods can really help to eliminate IBS symptoms in sorbitol intolerant patients.

Less common, but still occurring, is fructose intolerance, a condition in which some people have trouble digesting large amounts of fructose at once. Fructose is found in most fruits and many other whole foods. It's concentrated in fruit juices and dried fruits, which may be more problematic than fresh fruits. Fructose is especially a problem when it's mixed with sorbitol, as can happen in dietetic jams. Limiting your fruit servings to fresh, whole fruits instead of juices and avoiding foods that mix sorbitol and fructose may be useful for reducing IBS symptoms.

The good news is that simple dietary changes can help to alleviate symptoms of IBS. In many cases, high fiber foods may lessen IBS symptoms. Some excellent food sources of fiber include whole-grain breads and cereals, raspberries, mustard greens, turnip greens, collard greens, broccoli, cauliflower, and Swiss chard. It is important for people with IBS to increase their intake of fiber slowly, or symptoms can get temporarily worse before getting better. It's also very important when increasing fiber to also increase your water intake so that stools remain soft and easy to pass.

Yogurt is another potential addition to an IBS-friendly diet since it contains the bacteria lactobacillus acidophilus, the enzyme needed to digest lactose. It's important to look for yogurts that specifically say they contain live culture, as many types of yogurts are heat-treated to kill the bacteria before being sold. For people who either can't tolerate dairy or who choose not to eat dairy there are a number of very tasty soy-based yogurts.

Just worth mentioning, chamomile, ginger, and peppermint are also known to lessen the symptoms of IBS. Chamomile can be taken as a tea, or as a capsule. Ginger may be taken as a tea, a capsule, or even in food (such as Asian dishes) and ginger ale (be sure to check the label to ensure the product contains a significant amount of real ginger). Peppermint oil can be taken in either capsule or tea form. While they are most effective, capsules may cause anal irritation.

77

Lactose Intolerance Diet

Lactose intolerance is the inability to digest significant amounts of lactose, the predominant sugar of milk. This inability results from a shortage of the enzyme lactase, which breaks down lactose so it can be absorbed into the bloodstream. When the body does not produce enough lactase, lactose cannot be digested, which may result in lactose intolerance. A simple test done in your doctor's office can help determine whether or not lactose intolerance is a problem for you.

Common symptoms include nausea, cramps, bloating, gas, and diarrhea, which begin about 30 minutes to two hours after eating or drinking foods containing lactose. The severity of symptoms varies depending on the amount of lactose each individual can tolerate.

If you are lactose intolerant, you share this condition with many people. Between 30 and 50 million Americans are lactose intolerant. Certain ethnic and racial populations are more widely affected than others. As many as 75% of all African Americans and American Indians as well as 90% of Asian Americans are lactose intolerant. The condition is least common among persons of northern European descent.

People who have trouble digesting lactose can create their own lactose-intolerant diet by learning which dairy products and other foods they can eat without discomfort and which ones they should avoid. Many lactose intolerant sufferers can enjoy milk, ice cream, and other such products if they take them in small amounts or eat other food at the same time. Other lactose intolerant sufferers who react to very small amounts of lactose or have trouble limiting their intake of foods that contain lactose can use dietary supplements like lactase enzymes. Lactase is available without a prescription to help people digest foods that contain lactose. Lactase can be taken as tablets or liquid just before eating dairy food. Also, lactose-reduced dairy products are available at most supermarkets.

Unfortunately, lactose is found in a wide variety of food products such as milk, cheese, yogurt, and ice cream. It may also be hidden in foods such as baked goods, breakfast drink mixes, breakfast cereals, instant potatoes, soups, margarine, breads, non-kosher lunchmeats, salad dressings, candies and other snacks, "non-dairy" creamers and whipped toppings, pancake and cake mixes, powdered meal-replacement supplements, and some over-the-counter and prescription medications.

Smart shoppers learn to read food labels with care, looking not only for milk and lactose among the contents, but also for such words as whey, curds, milk by-products, dry milk solids, and nonfat dry milk powder. If any of these are listed on a label, the product contains lactose.

78

Menopause Diet

Menopause is the medical term for the end of a woman's menstrual periods. It is a natural part of aging, and occurs when the ovaries stop making hormones called estrogens. This causes estrogen levels to drop, and leads to the end of monthly menstual periods. This usually happens between the ages of 45 and 60, but it can happen earlier. Menopause can also occur when the ovaries are surgically removed or stop functioning for any other reason.

There is no way to prevent menopause. All women will experience it, but it is possible to minimize the problems and medical complications that often accompany it by combining a sensible diet with regular exercise. Taking this approach will lessen the risk of osteoporosis, heart disease, and stroke, while weight gain, depression, anxiety, hot flashes, and sleep disturbance can be reduced to a manageable level, and sometimes even eliminated.

No one knows what constitutes the optimum menopause diet. Each woman responds to menopause in her own unique way. But here are some general dietary guidelines to help maintain health and weight.

The basis of your diet should be a low-fat high-fiber diet including complex carbohydrates, a moderate amount of protein, sufficient essential fats, minimum saturated fats and cholesterol, and plenty of water. Since menopause puts women at increased risk of developing osteoporosis and heart disease, a well-planned balanced diet is particularly important at this time of life.

Fruits such as melons and bananas, and citrus fruits like oranges and lemons, are highly recommended; they are high in potassium and balance sodium and water retention. People should also include dried fruit such as apricots and figs. Vegetables including yams, collard greens, spinach, bok choi, broccoli, and cabbage may also make menopause more pleasant. Fruits and vegetables are good sources of vitamins and minerals, and the major sources of dietary fiber. Include soybeans, lentils, brown rice, and whole grains, and wheat germ. Seaweed such as Nori, Wakame, Kombu, and Arame contain natural hormones and plant chemicals that help during menopause. Oily fish like salmon, mackerel, sardines, herring, tuna, and trout are good since they are rich in omega-3 essential fatty acids. Soy products like calcium-fortified soy milk, and yogurt and tofu are also beneficial. Include canola and flaxseed oil, unsalted nuts like walnuts, Brazil nuts, and almonds, and seeds like sunflower, linseeds, and pumpkin seeds.

Plants contain phytoestrogens, estrogen-like compounds that mimic human estrogen. Simply put, phytoestrogens may trick your body into thinking it has more estrogen than it really does—potentially diminishing some of the discomforts caused by lower estrogen levels during menopause. Phytoestrogens are also found in soybeans, and it is thought that because Japanese eat a lot of soybeans, they suffer less severe menopausal symptoms than their Western counterparts.

Soy foods contain antioxidants, essential fatty acids, calcium, fiber, and carotenoids and flavonoids, all of which assist good diet nutrition, especially in menopause. Soy protein products can be good substitutes for animal products because, unlike some other beans, soy offers a "complete" protein profile.

It is important to avoid eating a diet that is high in fat, especially saturated fat. High-fat foods are usually high in calories and low in nutrients, exactly the opposite of what a woman in or past menopause needs. But it's even more important to get the right fats in your diet—fats that may protect against heart disease and cancer. Research indicates the right fats are omega-3 fatty acids that are not only found in fish but also in olive oil and canola oil. The wrong fats are saturated fats and trans-fatty acids found in foods like packaged cookies, chips, and crackers.

Vitamins and minerals are vital in any diet, but can be particularly beneficial during menopause. Calcium is essential for maintaining bone density, which tends to drop due to estrogen deficiency. Unfortunately, most women don't get enough calcium. A healthy pre-menopausal woman should have about 1,000 mgs of calcium per day, but women after menopause women should consume 1,500 mgs per day if they are not using a hormonal replacement, or 1,000 mgs per day in conjunction with hormonal replacement. Foods high in calcium include milk, yogurt, cheese and other dairy products; oysters, sardines, and canned salmon with bones; and dark-green leafy vegetables like spinach and broccoli. Vitamin D is needed for the absorption of calcium, and can be taken as a supplement. However, high doses of vitamin D can cause kidney stones, constipation, or abdominal pain, particularly in women with existing kidney problems. Coffee seems to interfere with calcium and bone-building. Vitamin E has been reported to relieve hot flashes, as well as being thought to help prevent heart attacks, Alzheimer's disease, and cancer. It is found in polyunsaturated vegetable oils, nuts, and seeds. Vitamin B2 is found in liver, kidney, mushrooms, and soybeans and has been shown to relieve menopausal headaches. Vitamin B6 may help alleviate depression, as well as protecting against heart disease and osteoporosis, and can be found in whole grains, bananas, nuts, and seeds. Vitamin B12 and folic acid might help with depression. Vitamin B12 can be obtained from liver, cheese, eggs, and fish. The mineral boron is another beneficial element of fruits and vegetables. Boron seems to increase the body's ability to hold onto estrogen. It also helps keep our bones strong by decreasing the amount of calcium we excrete each day.

79

Migraine Headache Diet

Migraine headaches are a common neurological disorder described as an intense throbbing or pounding pain felt in the forehead/temple, ear/jaw, or around the eyes. Classic migraines start on one side of the head, but may eventually spread to the other side. Other symptoms of classic migraines include speech difficulty, confusion, mood changes, fatigue, and unusual retention of fluid. An attack may last one to two pain-racked days and may occur several times a week, or rarely, as seldom once every few years.

Both men and women are affected by migraines, but the condition is most common in adult women. Both sexes may develop migraines in infancy, but most often the disorder begins between the ages of five and 35.

Some things can trigger a migraine or make it worse.

- Stress and time pressure, major hassles, major losses, anger, and conflict
- Smells and fumes, tobacco smoke, light glare or dazzle, weather changes
- Monthly periods, birth control pills, and estrogen therapy
- Too much, too little, or interrupted sleep
- Excessive activity
- Certain medicines may cause migraines
- Hunger, fasting, specific foods or beverages

The list of foods, food additives, and beverages that can precipitate headaches in migraine-susceptible persons is long and includes the following:

- Aged or strong cheese
- Citrus fruits
- Fatty or fried foods
- Chocolate
- Monosodium glutamate (MSG), which is found in Chinese food, Accent seasoning, Lawry's Seasoned Salt, canned soups, TV dinners, processed meats, and some processed nuts and snack chips

- Food dyes, food containing nitrites and nitrates (such as hot dogs, and salami), vegetable extracts, and some over-the-counter medicines
- Ice cream, sour cream, and yogurt (Some people are sensitive to all dairy products.)
- Meat, pork, and seafood
- Canned figs, bananas, raisins, broad beans, onions, and tomatoes
- Caffeine in coffee, tea, and sodas
- Alcoholic drinks, especially red wine, brandy, and whisky
- Vinegar and pickled foods such as pickled herring
- Smoked foods
- Nuts and peanuts
- Yeast-containing products such as fresh breads and doughnuts
- Saccharin or aspartame in diet foods or diet drinks
- Sulfites in shrimp and processed potatoes (like boxed mashed potato mix)

80

Pregnancy Diet

As you gain weight during pregnancy, it's tempting to diet—but don't do it. Nourishing a healthy, growing baby is your responsibility, and an imbalanced diet can be harmful to you and your baby. So forget the high carbo-hydrates/low-fat diet or the high fat/no carbohydrate diet or the liquid diet or the supplements. The main rule of healthy eating during pregnancy is having a balanced diet. This means your diet should include whole-grain products, vegetables, fruits, protein foods, and milk products as well as lots of hydrating fluids. To get the nutrients you and your baby need, choose the following foods every day.

- Whole grain products, which provide carbohydrates, your body's main source of energy.

- Fruits and vegetables, which provide important vitamins and minerals, as well as fiber to aid digestion.

- Protein foods such as meat, fish, and dried beans, are crucial for your baby's growth.

- If you are a vegetarian, be sure to eat eggs, tofu, and other soy products, dried beans and nuts, as well as a wide variety of grains every day.

- Milk products (including calcium-fortified soy milk), which helps build your baby's bones and teeth. If you have trouble digesting lactose, lactose-reduced milk products and calcium-fortified orange juice can help you get enough calcium.

Limit the amount of fat that you eat to no more than 30% (lower is better) of your daily calories using high-fat foods (such as butter, sour cream, salad dressings, and gravies) sparingly.

A vegetarian diet is safe as long as you take supplements (such as vitamin B12, folic acid, iron, zinc, magnesium, calcium, and vitamin D) to get the nutrients you need.

You also need to drink plenty of healthy fluids—six to eight cups a day. While water is best, you do get some water from juice. But keep in mind that juice is high in calories, while water has none.

Vitamins and Minerals

Most healthcare providers recommend that pregnant women take a pre-natal multivitamin containing the recommended amounts of vitamins, including folic acid. When taken before pregnancy and in the early weeks of pregnancy, adequate amounts of folic acid may help reduce the risk of birth defects of the brain and spinal cord. Natural sources of folic acid include orange juice, green leafy vegetables, beans, peanuts, broccoli, asparagus, peas, lentils, and enriched grain products. Iron is also very important with the need for iron doubling during pregnancy. Your healthcare provider may recommend a calcium supplement if you're unable to consume dairy products.

Coffee, Tea, and Alcoholic Beverages

Caffeine and alcohol actually prevent absorption of folic acid and iron—two essential nutrients during pregnancy—and pull calcium out of your bones, not to mention that they also directly affect the fetus and can have long-term developmental effects. Women who drink heavily during pregnancy can have a baby with a group of birth defects called fetal alcohol syndrome (FAS). FAS is the leading preventable cause of mental retardation. Some herbal teas should be avoided during pregnancy such as raspberry tea, cohash, slippery elm, ginseng, and green tea, which may stimulate contractions.

Uncooked or Cured Meats

Raw meats and eggs are risky during pregnancy because of the bacteria they may carry. So stay away from procciutto, runny eggs, shrimp cocktails, and ceviche.

Food Additives

Most additives are safe during pregnancy. However, there are a few additives that should be avoided, such as:

- MSG – Monosodium glutamate is a flavor enhancer in bouillon and Asian foods that can cause headaches and stomach upset.

- Nitrites – Nitrites are used to preserve meats, such as salami, frankfurters, luncheon meats, and smoked fish.

- Artificial food colorings – Colorings are in many processed foods, and most are considered safe during pregnancy. The ones to avoid are blue 1, blue 2, green 3, red 3, and yellow 6.

- Olestra (Olean) – Olestra hasn't been tested thoroughly enough to be considered safe during pregnancy.

- Saccharin – Saccharin has not been shown to be safe in pregnancy.

Premenstrual Syndrome Diet

Premenstrual syndrome (PMS) is actually a group of symptoms related to the menstrual cycle. PMS symptoms typically are bloating, breast tenderness, headaches, depression, lethargy, and irritability. The symptoms usually go away after the period starts. PMS may interfere with normal activities at home, school, or work. Of the estimated 40 million sufferers in the U.S., more than 5 million require medical treatment for marked mood and behavioral changes. Menopause, when monthly periods stop, brings an end to PMS. One way of managing PMS, or reducing the symptoms of PMS, is to make changes in your diet.

Foods That You Should Eat

Fiber-rich foods are particularly important in maintenance or restoration of healthy estrogen levels. The best sources of fiber are whole grains, legumes, root and leafy vegetables, fresh fruits, nuts, and seeds. Cruciferous vegetables, in particular, contain an important substance called indole-3-carbinol (I3C), a compound that can actually alter estrogen metabolism in a positive manner. Some examples of cruciferous vegetables include arugula, bok choi, broccoli, Brussels sprouts, cabbage, cauliflower, Chinese cabbage, collard greens, daikon, kale, kohlrabi, mustard greens, radishes, rutabaga, turnips, and watercress. Melons, bananas, and citrus fruits such as oranges, grapefruits, and lemons are particularly good because they are high in potassium. Potassium-rich foods help balance sodium and water retention.

Dietary fats should include the essential fatty acids and can be obtained from various natural oils and oil-containing foods. Good dietary sources of omega-6 fatty acids include cereals, eggs, poultry, most vegetable oils, whole-grain breads, baked goods, and margarine. Omega-3 fatty acids are found primarily in oily fish, such as salmon, lake trout, mackerel, tuna, and herring.

Foods To Avoid

Some women who suffer from PMS have a craving for food, especially for sweets. It satisfies their hunger and boosts their mood by increasing their sugar levels. But after eating this sugar they experience headaches, palpitations, or fatigue. Chocolate should be avoided since it aggravates mood swings and behavior changes. Studies have shown symptom-free women consume far less sugar and refined carbohydrates than those with symptoms.

Other foods to be avoided are coffee, tea, alcohol, and tobacco. Caffeine suppresses the neurotransmitter adenosine, which in turn calms nerve receptors. Without adenosine, nerve receptors can become overly reactive, leading to irritability, mood swings, and a worsening of symptoms.

Foods that are oily, fried, or spicy are to be avoided. Likewise eating a lot of meat is not advisable during these days. Studies have shown low-fat diets reduce estrogen levels, menstrual pain, and other premenstrual symptoms such as emotional changes and bloating. Also, PMS symptoms were lessened, and many women experienced significant relief, especially with water retention and concentration. Women who are losing too much blood, however, may need meat to help maintain iron levels.

Limiting salt may lessen bloating and water retention. One study found that restricting salt does not alleviate bloating or other symptoms, but salt reduction in the study was modest and may have been too small to affect improvement.

Vitamins and Minerals

An adequate vitamin and mineral intake may also help with PMS symptoms.

Vitamin B1: Studies have reported vitamin B1 (thiamin) as being effective in relieving cramps. Thiamin is found in almost all foods, with the highest concentration in pork. Other good sources of thiamin are dried fortified cereals, oatmeal, and sunflower seeds.

Vitamin B6: Vitamin B6 (pyridoxine) dietary supplementation will help patients with PMS. Typically, women take 100 mg per day, although one study suggested that a lower dose (50 mg) may have the same effect. Food sources of B6 are meats, oily fish, poultry, whole grains, dried fortified cereals, soybeans, avocados, baked potatoes with skins, watermelon, plantains, bananas, peanuts, and brewer's yeast.

Vitamin E: Several randomized controlled trials have shown that vitamin E may improve both physical and emotional symptoms. Studies do not agree about how much vitamin E may be helpful, but 300–400 IU per day is a safe dose that may be of benefit. It should be noted that vitamin E, like other antioxidants, may have damaging effects in high doses.

Calcium: Calcium can reduce the menstrual pain and the premenstrual tension. Some women get relief by being careful to take at least 1,200 mg of calcium per day through a combination of normal eating and taking supplements. Calcium-rich foods include dairy products, dark green vegetables, nuts, grains, beans, and canned salmon and sardines (including bones).

Magnesium: Most studies that have evaluated magnesium have failed to show overall benefit. One study of magnesium (200 mg/day) with 50 mg of vitamin B6 showed a significant reduction in anxiety symptoms compared to magnesium alone. Food sources of magnesium include nuts, legumes, whole grains, dark green vegetables, seafood (oysters), and meats.

82

Prostate Diet

The prostate gland, as part of the male reproductive system, secretes prostatic fluid, which contributes to the makeup of seminal fluid. A high proportion of men from middle age on have urinary problems associated with an enlarged prostate. Prostate enlargement of the gland is not prostate cancer, nor does it increase one's chances of developing prostate cancer. An enlarged prostate can raise PSA (prostate-specific antigen) levels to two or three times the normal level. High PSA levels do, however, carry a higher chance of having cancer.

Inflammation of the prostate gland is known as prostatitis. If the prostate grows too large it may constrict the urethra and impede the flow of urine, making urination difficult, painful and in extreme cases, completely impossible.

Overall, it seems that levels of saturated fat in the diet can greatly increase the risk of prostate cancer. Saturated fats have been related to cancer in many studies, and saturated fats from animal products seem to be implicated most significantly. Therefore, making sure you have a healthy diet and keeping your intake of fat in check can help to prevent or decrease the risk of prostate cancer. Dairy products have also been linked to prostate cancer because of their saturated fat content. As an added bonus, reducing your consumption of fat can also decrease the risk of other cancers, as well as diseases such as heart disease and diabetes.

It is also widely accepted that consuming plenty of fruit and vegetables can help to prevent cancers because of the antioxidants they contain. It is recommended that you eat at least five portions of fruits and vegetables every day.

Preventative Measures
- Eat a diet low in fat and, in particular, low in saturated fat.
- Include plenty of fruit and vegetables in your day-to-day diet.
- Avoid or decrease your intake of alcohol, coffee, beer (particularly after dinner), and tobacco.

- Increase intake of foods rich in omega-3 fatty acids (cold-water fish—salmon, sardines, and mackerel) and in zinc. (raw pumpkin seeds for omega-3 and zinc).

- Eat foods containing calcium (that is particularly important for men with advancing prostate cancer).

- Maintain a healthy body weight by balancing physical activity and food intake.

83

Type 2 Diabetes Diet

Type 2 diabetes is the most common form of diabetes. In Type 2 diabetes, either the body does not produce enough insulin, or the cells ignore the insulin. After a meal, food is broken down into a sugar called glucose, which is carried by the blood to cells throughout the body. Cells use the insulin to help them process blood glucose into energy. When glucose builds up in the blood, instead of being used by the cells, it can cause two problems:

- Right away, your cells may be starved for energy.
- Over time, high blood glucose levels may hurt your eyes, kidneys, nerves, or heart.

Type 2 diabetes may account for up to 95% of all diagnosed cases of diabetes, and is increasingly being diagnosed in children and adolescents. Individuals who are physically inactive and/or overweight are much more likely to develop Type 2 diabetes. Overweight people are twice as likely to develop Type 2 diabetes as are people who are not overweight. For obese men, the risk of developing diabetes is 40 times higher than for men who have a healthy weight, and for obese women the risk more than doubles. Similarly, people who move from a non-Westernized country to a Westernized country increase their risk for Type 2 diabetes considerably. Studies suggest that moderate, regular exercise such as walking for 30 minutes most days of the week, is enough to protect against the development of diabetes.

People who have Type 2 diabetes have the potential to reduce the harmful effects of diabetes purely by making some changes to their lifestyle. People who have Type 2 diabetes should meet with a registered dietitian or a physician to plan an individualized diet within the general guidelines that takes into consideration their own health needs. There is no single diet that meets all the needs of everyone with Type 2 diabetes. In addition to a regular balanced diet, effective diabetic-management requires a healthy regular lifestyle, which should include regular exercise and sensible weight control.

The American Diabetes Association (ADA) recommends that individuals with diabetes consume a healthy, low-fat diet, rich in grains, fruits, and vegetables. Meal planning also includes eating the right amount of food and eating meals at the right time. The ADA currently recommends that 50 to 60% of a person's diet should come from carbohydrates, 10 to 20% from lean sources of protein, and less than 30% from fats. Avoid saturated fats (found in animal products) and trans-fatty acids (hard margarines, commercial products, and fast foods). In selecting fats or oils, prefer monounsaturated fats (virgin olive oil, canola oil), although also include polyunsaturated oils as well (sunflower, rapeseed). Different studies have reported an association between Type 2 diabetes and both saturated fats and trans-fatty acids. Diabetics who eat healthy, well-balanced diets will not need to take extra vitamins or minerals to treat their condition.

The most important dietary consideration for people with Type 2 diabetes is the need to control their blood sugar levels. The most common method for controlling blood sugar is the use of the Diabetic Exchange Lists. The objective of the exchange lists is to maintain the proper balance of carbohydrates, proteins, and fats throughout the day. More sophisticated methods include counting carbohydrate grams and using the glycemic index to determine the impact of carbohydrates on blood sugar.

Carbohydrate foods have the greatest direct effect on blood glucose levels. Carbohydrates are broken down into glucose by digestive enzymes. The glucose is then absorbed from the intestine into the bloodstream (usually 1–2 hours after eating) and this causes the blood glucose level to rise after a meal. However, proteins and fats in the diet do affect blood glucose levels too.

People with Type 2 diabetes do not produce enough insulin to cope with the sharp rise in blood glucose that happens after a meal. Therefore choosing the right carbohydrates that are more slowly digested can reduce the "post-meal spike" in blood glucose, which in turn reduces the demand on the beta cells for insulin.

Different types of carbohydrate foods are digested at different rates and therefore have different effects in terms of raising the blood glucose level after a meal. Some foods are quite rapidly digested to glucose while others take longer for the glucose to hit the bloodstream. The effect of different carbohydrate foods on blood glucose levels has been quantified by the glycemic index (GI). Foods with a low GI cause less of a spike in post-meal blood glucose than those with a high GI.

Choose whole grains and whole-grain products over highly processed carbohydrates. Refined carbohydrates such as white bread, white rice, mashed potatoes, doughnuts, bagels, and many breakfast cereals have a high GI. That means they cause sustained spikes in blood sugar and insulin levels. Complex carbohydrates such as whole wheat, brown rice, other whole grains, most beans and nuts, and whole-grain breakfast cereals that aren't as easily digested cause lower, slower increases in blood sugar and insulin. Such foods have a low GI.

The most significant effect of fat on blood glucose levels is probably to slow down the rise in blood glucose after a meal. There are different types of fats—some can be beneficial to our health, but others can increase the risk of high blood pressure and heart disease. Too much saturated fat and cholesterol in the diet can result in unhealthy levels of blood fats. However, monounsaturated fats may improve your lipid profile.

Excess protein in the diet that is not needed by the body is converted to glucose by the liver. This means that consuming large amounts of protein can result in an increase in blood glucose levels several hours after eating.

SECTION III

Diets by Health & Government Organizations

American Cancer Society

The American Cancer Society recommends a predominantly plant-based diet that includes a variety of vegetables, fruits, and grain-based foods for nutrition and prevention for certain types of cancers.

The Society recommends limiting consumption of meats, especially high-fat meats. Foods from animal sources remain major contributors of total fat, saturated fat, and cholesterol in the American diet. Although meats are good sources of high-quality protein and supply many important vitamins and minerals, consumption of meat—especially red meats—has been linked to cancers, most notably colon and prostate cancers.

The Society recommends limiting consumption of alcohol since alcoholic beverages, along with cigarette smoking, cause cancers of the oral cavity, esophagus, and larynx. Cancer risk increases with the amount of alcohol consumed and may start to rise with the intake of as few as two drinks per day.

The Society also recommends at least 30 minutes of moderate physical activity on most days of the week since physical activity can help protect against some cancers.

American Heart Association

The American Heart Association (AHA) publishes dietary guidelines for general heart health. The AHA emphasizes a diet rich in fruits, vegetables, legumes (beans), whole grains, low-fat dairy products, fish, lean meats, and poultry.

Fruits and vegetables are high in nutrients and fiber, and are relatively low in calories. Choose five or more servings per day of fruits and vegetables. Dark green, deep orange, or yellow fruits and vegetables are especially nutritious. People whose diet includes a high intake of fruits and vegetables are found to be associated with a lower risk of developing heart disease, stroke, and hypertension. AHA recommends whole-grain products because they provide complex carbohydrates, vitamins, minerals, and fiber. Dietary patterns high in grain products and fiber have been associated with decreased risk of cardiovascular disease.

The AHA stresses the importance of achieving and maintaining a desirable blood cholesterol level by limiting foods high in saturated fat, cholesterol, and trans-fatty acids. Trans-fatty acids are fats found in foods that contain partially hydrogenated vegetable oils including packaged cookies, crackers, and other baked goods, commercially prepared fried foods, some margarine, and the oil used to fry foods in most restaurants and fast-food chains. Many foods high in saturated fat are also high in cholesterol. Saturated fat should not exceed 10% of total calories; daily cholesterol should not exceed 300 mg. People with elevated LDL (bad) cholesterol levels or existing cardiovascular disease should not get more than 7% of their total calories from saturated fat and should only consume 200 mg a day or less of cholesterol. For people with risk factors for heart disease or those who already have heart disease, further reduction in saturated fat intake is recommended. Include fat-free and low-fat milk products, fish, legumes (beans), skinless poultry, and lean meats. Eating fruits and low-fat dairy products also helps to keep saturated fat levels low.

The AHA dietary guidelines also recommend eating fish, because a growing body of evidence indicates that omega-3 fatty acids may protect the heart. Experts continue to discourage the use of omega-3 fatty acids from fish oil capsules because their use has demonstrated no long-term benefits.

Limit your intake of foods high in calories or low in nutrition, including foods like soft drinks and candy that have a lot of sugars. Eat less than 6 grams of salt (sodium chloride) per day (2,400 milligrams of sodium). Limit alcohol intake to no more than two drinks per day for men, and one drink per day for women.

Maintain a level of physical activity that keeps you fit and matches the number of calories you eat. Walk or do other activities for at least 30 minutes on most days. If you need to lose weight consume fewer calories than your body burns.

The Association still recommends that individuals get their nutrients from foods, not supplements.

86

Harvard School of Public Health

As an alternative to the USDA's food pyramid, faculty members in the Harvard School of Public Health built the Healthy Eating Pyramid. It resembles the USDA's in shape, but takes into consideration, and puts into perspective, the wealth of research conducted during the last 10 years that has reshaped the definition of healthy eating. The Healthy Eating Pyramid sits on a foundation of daily exercise and weight control, and builds from there recommending whole-grain foods and plant oils as the next tier, with vegetables and fruits on the following tier, and working its way up the pyramid with nuts and legumes; fish, poultry and eggs; and dairy or calcium supplements. At the top of the pyramid are red meat and butter, along with white rice, white bread, potatoes, pasta, and sweets.

Whole-Grain Foods (at most meals)

The body needs carbohydrates mainly for energy. The best sources of carbohydrates are whole grains such as oatmeal, whole-wheat bread, and brown rice. The body can't digest whole grains as quickly as it can highly processed carbohydrates (e.g., white flour and white rice). The slower digestion keeps blood sugar and insulin levels in check rather than rising, then falling too quickly, as in the case with highly processed carbohydrates.

Plant Oils

The Healthy Food Pyramid places a lot of importance on plant oils since the average American gets one third or more of their daily calories from fats. Good sources of healthy unsaturated fats include olive, canola, soy, corn, sunflower, peanut, and other vegetable oils, as well as fatty fish such as salmon.

Vegetables (in abundance) and Fruits (two to three times)

Eating plenty of fruits and vegetables can help you ward off heart disease and stroke, control blood pressure and cholesterol, prevent some types of cancer, avoid painful intestinal ailments, and guard against cataract and macular degeneration, two common causes of vision loss.

Fish, Poultry, and Eggs (zero to two times)

Fish, poultry, and eggs are all important sources of protein. Eating fish can reduce the risk of heart disease and poultry is low in saturated fat. Although eggs have a bad reputation because they contain fairly high levels of cholesterol, they're not that harmful if eaten in moderation and are a good source of protein.

Nuts and Legumes (one to three times)

Nuts and legumes are other excellent sources of protein as well as fiber, vitamins, and minerals. Legumes include black beans, navy beans, garbanzos, and other beans that are usually sold dried. Nuts include almonds, walnuts, pecans, peanuts, hazelnuts, and pistachios. Many kinds of nuts contain healthy fats and are good for your heart.

Dairy or Calcium Supplement (one to two times)

Although dairy products have traditionally been Americans' main source of calcium the Healthy Food Pyramid recommends no-fat or low-fat dairy products or calcium supplements.

Red Meat and Butter (Use Sparingly)

The Healthy Food Pyramid recommends eating red meat and butter sparingly because they contain lots of saturated fat. Try substituting fish or chicken for red meat as much as possible, as well as olive oil for butter.

White Rice, White Bread, Potatoes, Pasta, and Sweets (Use Sparingly)

White rice, white bread, potatoes, pasta, and sweets can cause a rapid increase in blood sugar that can lead to weight gain, diabetes, heart disease, and other chronic disorders. As mentioned, eating whole-grain carbohydrates keeps blood sugar and insulin levels in check.

Multiple Vitamins

The Healthy Food Pyramid recommends taking a daily multivitamin as a nutritional backup.

Alcohol (in moderation)

The Healthy Food Pyramid recommends drinking alcohol only in moderation, since alcohol has risks as well as benefits. For men, a good balance point is one to two drinks a day. For women, it's at most one drink a day.

87

National Heart, Lung and Blood Institute

The DASH diet (short for Dietary Approaches to Stop Hypertension) is designed by the National Heart, Lung and Blood Institute to reduce high blood pressure (hypertension) and boost nutrition and general health. The DASH diet includes an abundance of fruits, vegetables, and low-fat dairy products while reducing your consumption of total fat, saturated fat, cholesterol, and sweets. It also is low in cholesterol, high in dietary fiber, potassium, calcium, and magnesium, and moderately high in protein.

While excessive sodium is not encouraged, it is not the sole focus of this dietary approach for managing high blood pressure. The DASH diet is also unique from other blood-pressure-reducing diets because it focuses more on things that you can eat and less on things you cannot eat.

The biggest component of the DASH diet, and perhaps the most challenging part for some people, is the increased fruit and vegetable requirements. The diet recommends more fruits and vegetables than most people are probably used to.

The DASH diet below is based on a 2,000-calorie-a-day meal plan. Check with your healthcare practitioner about whether the DASH diet may be the right diet for you.

Dash Eating Plan

Food Group	Servings*	Serving	Rich in...
Grains	7–8/day	1 slice bread; ½ cup cooked rice, pasta, or cereal	Energy and fiber
Vegetables	4–5/day	1 cup raw leafy vegetable; ½ cup cooked vegetable; 6 ounces vegetable juice	Potassium, magnesium, fiber

Food Group	Servings*	Serving	Rich in...
Fruits	4–5/day	1 medium fresh fruit 1/4 cup dried, frozen, or canned fruit	Potassium, magnesium, fiber
Low-fat dairy products	2–3/day	8 ounces milk; 1 cup yogurt; 1.5 ounces cheese	Calcium, protein
Meat, fish, poultry	2 or less/day	3 ounces lean cooked meat, poultry, fish; 1 egg	Magnesium, protein
Nuts, seeds, dried beans	4–5/week	½ cup cooked beans; 1.5 ounces or 1/3 cups nuts; 1/2 ounce or 2 tablespoons seeds	Energy, magnesium, protein, potassium, fiber
Fats and oils	2–3/day	1 teaspoon soft margarine 2 tablespoons light salad dressing 1 teaspoon vegetable oil	*In addition to fats added to foods, remember to choose foods low in fat.
Sweets	5/week	1 cup sweetened beverage ½ ounce candy 1 small piece of cake	Select low-fat sweets
* If your caloric needs are higher or lower, you may eat more or fewer servings accordingly.			

In addition to the eating plan shown above, there are a number of diet tips and healthy habits for controlling your blood pressure as follows.

- Choose whole grains over white flour or pasta products.

- Make changes gradually, since additional fruits, vegetables, and whole grains increase your fiber intake. Most people find it hard to change their diet if they try to change too much too soon. Make sure to also increase your fluid intake as you add more fiber to your diet.

- To meet your higher fruit and vegetable requirements, try adding vegetables to soup, omelets, and sandwiches, and enjoy fruit for dessert.

- Avoid saturated fat (although include calcium-rich dairy products that are no- or low-fat).

- When choosing fats, select monounsaturated oils such as olive or canola oils. Studies have reported a reduced need for anti-hypertension medication in people with a high intake of virgin olive oil, but not sunflower oil, a polyunsaturated fat.

- Try low-fat or fat-free condiments such as fat-free salad dressing. Salad dressings can be a huge source of fat, so you can substantially reduce your fat intake just by using fat-free salad dressing. Read food labels on margarines and salad dressings to choose those lowest in saturated fat and trans fat. Some margarines are now trans-fat free. Choose low-fat or fat-free dairy products to reduce your intake of saturated fat, total fat, cholesterol, and calories.

- Limit meat to six ounces a day (two servings).

- Choose modest amounts of protein (preferably fish, poultry, or soy products). Soy in combination with fiber-rich foods or supplements may have specific benefits. Oily fish may also be particularly beneficial. They contain omega-3 fatty acids, which have been associated with heart and nerve protection.

- Include nuts, seeds, or legumes (dried beans or peas) daily.

- Maintain a healthy weight.

- Increase your daily physical activity. A regular exercise routine (20–30 minutes, at least three times per week) can help lower blood pressure and aid in weight loss.

- Try to keep your daily sodium intake within 2,400 milligrams, the upper limit. Keep in mind that just one teaspoon of added table salt contains 2,000 milligrams of sodium.

- Increase calcium, potassium, and magnesium intake (these minerals are already built into the DASH diet.)

- Excessive alcohol consumption, more than one to two drinks per day, is not recommended. It may also increase your risk for having a stroke if you already have high blood pressure.

88

U.S. Government Dietary Guidelines

The U.S. Department of Agriculture (USDA) and the U.S. Department of Health and Human Services (DHHS) publish the *Dietary Guidelines for Americans* to help individuals meet nutrient requirements, promote health, support active lives, and reduce chronic disease risks. The Dietary Guidelines for Americans are the cornerstone of Federal nutrition policy and nutrition education activities. They are jointly issued by USDA and DHHS and updated every five years.

The intent of the Dietary Guidelines is to summarize and synthesize knowledge regarding individual nutrients and food components into recommendations for a pattern of eating that can be adopted by the public.

A basic premise of the Dietary Guidelines is that nutrient needs should be met primarily through consuming foods. Foods provide an array of nutrients and other compounds that may have beneficial effects on health. In certain cases, fortified foods and dietary supplements may be useful sources for one or more nutrients that otherwise might be consumed in less than recommended amounts. However, dietary supplements, while recommended in some cases, cannot replace a healthful diet.

The USDA Food Guide and the DASH (Dietary Approaches to Stop Hypertension) Eating Plan are two eating patterns that exemplify the Dietary Guidelines. These eating patterns are not weight loss diets, but rather illustrative examples of how to eat in accordance with the Dietary Guidelines.

The Dietary Guidelines use a 2,000-calorie level as a reference for consistency with the Nutritional Facts Panel.

The following is a summary of the Dietary Guidelines for 2005.

Adequate Nutrients within Calorie Needs

- Consume a variety of nutrient-dense foods and beverages within and among the basic food groups while choosing foods that limit the intake of saturated and trans-fatty acids, cholesterol, added sugars, salt, and alcohol.

- Meet recommended intakes within energy needs by adopting a balanced eating pattern, such as shown by the USDA Food Guide Pyramid.

Weight Management

- To maintain body weight in a healthy range, balance calories from foods and beverages with calories expended.

- To prevent gradual weight gain over time, make small decreases in food and beverage calories and increase physical activity.

Physical Activity

- Engage in regular physical activity and reduce sedentary activities to promote health, psychological well-being, and a healthy body weight.

- Achieve physical fitness by including cardiovascular conditioning, stretching exercises for flexibility, and resistance exercises or calisthenics for muscle strength.

Food Groups to Encourage

- Consume sufficient amount of fruits and vegetables while staying within energy needs. Two cups of fruit and 2.5 cups of vegetables per day are recommended.

- Choose a variety of fruits and vegetables each day. In particular, select from all five vegetable subgroups (dark green, orange, legumes, starchy vegetables, and others) several times a week.

- Consume three or more ounce-equivalents of whole-grain products per day, with the rest of the recommended grains coming from enriched or whole-grain products. In general, at least half the grains should come from whole grains.

- Consume three cups per day of fat-free or low-fat milk, or equivalent milk products.

Fats

- Consume less then 10% of calories from saturated fatty acids and less than 300 mg/day of cholesterol, and keep trans-fatty acid consumption as low as possible.

- Keep total fat intake between 20 and 35% of calories, with most fats coming from sources of polyunsaturated and monounsaturated fatty acids, such as fish, nuts, and vegetable oils.

- When selecting and preparing meat, poultry, dry beans, and milk or milk products, make choices that are lean, low-fat, or fat-free.

- Limit intake of fats and oils high in saturated and/or trans-fatty acids, and choose products low in such fats and oils.

Carbohydrates

- Choose fiber-rich fruits, vegetables, and whole grains often.

- Choose and prepare foods and beverages with little added sugars and caloric sweeteners, such amounts as suggested by the USDA Food Guide and the DASH Eating Plan.

Sodium and Potassium

- Consume less than 2,300 mg (approximately 1 teaspoon of salt) of sodium per day.

- Choose and prepare foods with little salt. At the same time, consume potassium-rich foods, such as fruits and vegetables.

Glossary

ACCEPTABLE DAILY INTAKE (ADI)—The amount of chemical that, if ingested daily over a lifetime, appears to be without appreciable effect.

ADDITIVES (FOOD ADDITIVES)—Any natural or synthetic material, other than the basic raw ingredients, used in the production of a food item to enhance the final product.

ALLERGEN—The part of a food (a protein) that stimulates the immune system of food allergic individuals. A single food can contain multiple food allergens. Carbohydrates or fats are not allergens.

ALLERGY—Any adverse reaction to an otherwise harmless food or food component (a protein) that involves the body's immune system. To avoid confusion with other types of adverse reactions to foods, it is important to use the terms "food allergy" or "food hypersensitivity" only when the immune system is involved in causing the reaction.

AMINO ACIDS—Amino acids function as the building blocks of proteins. There are 20 different amino acids the body uses from food to make various proteins. However, the body itself can make about 11 of these amino acids, leaving nine amino acids that we must get from food. These remaining nine are called "essential" amino acids, meaning it is essential that we get them from our diet.

ANEMIA—A condition in which a deficiency in the size or number of erythrocytes (red blood cells) or the amount of hemoglobin they contain limits the exchange of oxygen and carbon dioxide between the blood and the tissue cells. Most anemia is caused by a lack of nutrients required for normal erythrocyte synthesis, principally iron, vitamin B12, and folic acid.

ANOREXIZ NERVOSA—An eating disorder characterized by refusal to maintain a minimally normal weight for height and age.

ANTIOXIDANTS—Substances that may protect cells from the damage caused by unstable molecules known as free radicals. Antioxidants interact with and stabilize free radicals and may prevent some of the damage free radicals otherwise might cause. Antioxidants are found naturally in many foods, primarily fruits and vegetables. There are claims that antioxidants help prevent or reduce the effects of a variety of diseases, including cardiovascular disease, diabetes, Alzheimer's, and various forms of cancer.

ATHEROSCLEROSIS—A condition that exists when too much cholesterol builds up in the blood and accumulates in the walls of the blood vessels.

BETA-CAROTENE—Beta-carotene (also known a pro-vitamin A) is converted to vitamin A by the body. Beta-carotene is an antioxidant—a substance that protects the body against disease and premature aging by fighting the cell-damaging chemical called free radicals.

BODY MASS INDEX (BMI)—A calculation used for determining over-weight and obesity in adults by dividing a person's weight in kilograms by height in meters squared (BMI = $[kg/m^2]$. BMI can also be calculated in pounds and inches: BMI=$[lbs/in^2]$ X 703. The general guideline currently recommended by the Center for Disease Control and Prevention is that individuals with a BMI of 25 to 29.9 are considered overweight and those individuals with a BMI greater than 30 are considered obese.

BULIMIA NERVOSA—An eating disorder characterized by rapid con-sumption of a large amount of food in a short period of time, with a sense of lack of control during the episode and self-evaluation unduly influenced by body weight and shape. There are two forms of the condition: purging and non-purging. The first type regularly engages in purging through self-induced vomiting or the excessive use of laxatives or diuretics. Alterna-tively, the non-purging type controls weight through strict dieting, fasting or excessive exercise.

CAFFEINE—A naturally occurring substance found in the leaves, seeds, or fruits of over 63 plant species worldwide that is part of a group of com-pounds known as methylxanthines. The most commonly known sources of caffeine are coffee and cocoa beans, cola nuts, and tea leaves.

CALCIUM—A mineral that builds bones and strengthens bones, helps in muscle contraction and heartbeat, assists with nerve functions, and blood clotting. Milk and other dairy foods such as yogurt and most cheeses are the best sources of calcium. In addition, dark green leafy vegetables, fish with edible bones, and calcium-fortified foods supply significant amounts. Other good sources include tofu, chickpeas and other legumes, nuts and seeds (almonds, Brazil nuts, pistachios, sunflower seeds, sesame seeds, flax seed), dried fruit, figs, broccoli, and fortified soy- and rice-milk.

CALORIE—The amount of energy required to raise the temperature of one milliliter (ml) of water at a standard initial temperature by one degree centigrade (1°C). Fat and alcohol are high in calories.

CARBOHYDRATES—Carbohydrates are a critical source of fuel for your brain, red blood cells, and muscles providing four calories per gram. In the body, carbohydrates are broken down to glucose, which is used to generate energy. Not eating enough carbohydrates forces your body to make glucose from other body tissues, primarily muscle protein. In addition, fiber is a form of carbohydrate that aids intestinal health, can help lower cholesterol, and help manage blood sugar levels. Carbohydrates are found in sugars, fruits, vegetables, and cereals and grains. Meats generally do not have carbohydrates. In general, carbohydrates are either complex or simple. Simple carbohydrates are named so because they are made up of monosaccharides and disaccharides, which are "simple" molecules. Simple carbohydrates include sugar, high fructose corn syrup, and white flour and white rice to name a few. Complex carbohydrates are named so because they are made up of polysaccharides, which are much bigger, more "complex" molecules. Complex carbohydrates include whole-wheat flour, brown rice, and fruits, vegetables, grains, and beans in their natural forms.

CHOLESTEROL—A fat-like substance classified as a lipid that is vital to life. However, too much cholesterol in the blood can increase the risk of heart disease. Cholesterol is not only manufactured by your body, it also comes from the foods we eat, and is then known as dietary cholesterol. Animal products such as egg yolks, higher-fat milk products, poultry, shellfish, and meat are high in cholesterol—and also in saturated fats. Dietary cholesterol is found only in animal foods. Abundant in organ meats and egg yolks, cholesterol is also contained in meats, poultry, and shellfish. Vegetable oils are cholesterol-free.

Blood cholesterol is divided into three separate classes of lipoproteins: very-low density lipoprotein (VLDL); low-density lipoprotein (LDL), which contains most of the cholesterol found in the blood; and high-density lipoprotein (HDL). LDL is a cause in coronary heart disease and is popularly known as the "bad cholesterol." By contrast, HDL is increasingly considered desirable and known as the "good cholesterol."

DIABETES—A disease in which the body can no longer produce or properly use insulin, a hormone required to convert sugars and starches from the food we eat into the energy we need.

DIETARY GUIDELINES FOR AMERICANS—Guidelines for eating based on scientific consensus and forming the cornerstone of federal nutrition policy. The Dietary Guidelines are issued by the United States Department of Agriculture and the Department of Health and Human Services (USDA/DHHS) every five years.

EATING DISORDERS—Eating disorders may be classified as anorexia, bulimia, compulsive overeating, binge eating, or any combination of these. Each is based on specific diagnostic criteria.

ENRICHED FOODS—Enriched foods are those that nutrients have been added to replace the nutrients which were lost during food processing. For example, vitamin B is lost in processing wheat to white flour and is then added back to the flour.

ESSENTIAL FATTY ACIDS (EFAs)—Essential Fatty Acids are necessary fats that humans cannot synthesize, so they must be obtained through diet. EFAs are long-chain polyunsaturated fatty acids derived from linolenic, linoleic, and oleic acids. There are two families of EFAs: omega-3 and omega-6 fatty acids. Omega-9 is necessary yet "non-essential" because the body can manufacture a modest amount on its own, provided essential EFAs are present. Omega-3 fatty acids are derived from linolenic acid, omega-6 from linoleic acid, and omega-9 from oleic acid.

FATS—Fats are referred to in the plural because there is no one type of fat. Fats are a vital nutrient in a healthy diet. Fats supply essential fatty acids, such as linoleic acid, which is especially important to childhood growth. Fat helps maintain healthy skin and regulate cholesterol metabolism, and is a precursor of prostaglandins—hormone-like substances that regulate some body processes. Dietary fat is needed to carry fat-soluble vitamins A, D, E, and K and to aid in their absorption from the intestine. The building blocks of fat are called fatty acids. There are two main types of fats found in foods: unsaturated and saturated fats. Some fats can be beneficial to our health, but others can increase the risk of high blood pressure and heart disease. Too much saturated fat in the diet can result in unhealthy levels of cholesterol. Bad fats, such as trans fats, are found in margarines, packaged baked goods, fried foods in most fast-food restaurants, and any product that lists "partially hydrogenated vegetable oil" on the label. However, monounsaturated and polyunsaturated fats could help lower blood cholesterol levels. Good fats, such as the polyunsaturated fats, are found in tuna, salmon, liquid vegetable oils, and many nuts. Numerous health and government authorities, including the U.S. Surgeon General, the National Academy of Sciences, the American Heart Association, and the American Dietetic Association, recommend reducing dietary fat to 30% or less of total calories.

FERULIC ACID—A type of phenol found in various fruits, vegetables, and citrus fruits, which has antioxidant-like activities that may reduce the risk of degenerative diseases, heart disease, and eye disease.

FIBER—An important component of many complex carbohydrates. It is almost always found only in plants, particularly vegetables, fruits, whole grains, nuts, and legumes (dried beans, peanuts, and peas). Meats and dairy products do not contain fiber. Unlike other forms of carbohydrates, our bodies cannot digest fiber, which gives it unique health properties compared to other nutrients. Studies indicate that high-fiber diets can reduce the risks of heart disease and certain types of cancer. Although there are numerous types of fiber, the two main types are insoluble and soluble. Soluble fiber in cereals, oatmeal, beans, and other foods has been found to lower blood cholesterol. Insoluble fiber in cauliflower, cabbage, and other vegetables and fruits helps move foods through the stomach and intestine, thereby decreasing the risk of cancers of the colon and rectum.

FOOD GUIDE PYRAMID—A graphic design used to communicate the recommended daily food choices contained in the Dietary Guidelines for Americans. The information provided was developed and promoted by the U.S. Department of Agriculture and the U.S. Department of Health and Human Services.

FOOD LABELS—Every year thousands of new foods are introduced, many of them advertised as nutritionally beneficial. The current food labels show the number of calories from fat, the amount of nutrients that are potentially dangerous (fat, cholesterol, sodium, sugars) as well as useful nutrients (fiber, carbohydrates, protein, vitamins). Labels also show "daily values," the percentage of a daily diet that each of the important nutrients offers in a single serving. Unfortunately, the daily value is based on 2,000 calories, generally much higher than most people should eat.

FOOD PRESERVATIVES—Ingredients added to foods. All preservatives prevent spoilage either by slowing the growth of organisms that live on food or by protecting the food from oxygen.

FORTIFIED FOODS—Fortified foods have nutrients added to them that were not present originally. For example, milk is fortified with vitamin D, which helps your body absorb the calcium and phosphorus found naturally in milk.

FRUCTOSE—A monosaccharide found naturally in fruits, as an added sugar in a crystalline form, and as a component of high-fructose corn syrup (HFCS).

GLYCEMIC INDEX (GI)—A measure of how quickly a particular food's carbohydrates are converted into glucose (blood sugar). Some simple sugars, like table sugar, will enter the bloodstream slower than many complex carbohydrates, such as whole-grain bread and brown rice. The faster a carbohydrate enters the bloodstream, the higher its glycemic index. The higher the glycemic index of a carbohydrate, the greater the increase in insulin levels. Fruits and vegetables tend to have a low glycemic index, whereas white breads, pasta, white rice, and starches tend to have a high glycemic index. Dieters should focus on eating carbohydrates that have a low impact on blood sugar levels, which leads to steadier blood sugar levels and potentially improved appetite control.

GLYCEMIC LOAD (GL)—Measures both quality and quantity of carbohydrates by looking at a food's GI and adjusting that figure to reflect a realistic serving size. For example, carrots have a relatively high glycemic index, but the total amount of carbohydrates in a serving of carrots is very low, so carrots have a low Glycemic Load.

GLUCOSE—The only simple carbohydrate that circulates in the bloodstream. Glucose is the primary fuel used by the brain. It can also be stored in the liver and muscles in a polymer form known as glycogen. Glucose comes from grape juice, honey, and certain vegetables, among other things.

HIGH DENSITY PROTEIN (HDL)—The "good" cholesterol that helps remove cholesterol from cells. If insulin levels go up, then HDL levels go down. The lower your HDL level, the more likely you are to suffer cardiovascular complications.

HYDROGENATED FATS—Unsaturated fats can be made more saturated (and therefore harder at room temperature) by a process called hydrogenation. Hydrogenation is done to increase the shelf life of fats and to change how hard they are at room temperature. (Harder fats make crispier crackers and better pie crusts, and they are easier to spread on toast.) Hydrogenation changes unsaturated fats into more saturated fats that can raise blood cholesterol. Furthermore, during the hydrogenation process, some unnatural bonds, called trans bonds, are formed, which also negatively affect blood cholesterol. Sometimes called "trans fats," these hydrogenated fats are as harmful for your health as saturated fats.

INSOLUBLE FIBER—A type of dietary fiber found in wheat bran, cauliflower, cabbage, and other vegetables and fruits that helps move foods through the digestive system and thereby decreasing the risks of cancers of the colon and rectum. Insoluble fiber may also help reduce the risk of breast cancer. Of special note, nuts, such as almonds, macadamia, and walnuts may be highly heart protective, independent of their fiber content.

IRON—Iron is necessary for the development of hemoglobin and is used in protein metabolism. Collards, kale, broccoli, and other dark greens are good iron sources, as are dried fruits, whole grains, nuts, seeds, beans, and legumes. Iron absorption is increased when a source of ascorbic acid (vitamin C) such as dark leafy vegetables, tomatoes, or citrus is served along with the iron-rich food.

MINERALS—Simple chemical elements that are an essential part of the body's functioning.

MONOUNSATURATED FATS—Type of fat found in many foods but predominantly in avocados and canola oil, olive oil, and peanut oil. Studies suggest that monounsaturated fat tends to lower LDL cholesterol levels.

MONO- AND DI-GLYCERIDES—Emulsifying agents found in shortening, margarine, cacao products, and bakery products. Usually derived from soybean fat, these food additives keep food products from separating.

MSG (MONOSODIUM GLUTAMATE)—The sodium salt of glutamic acid, or glutamate, one of the most common amino acids found in nature.

OBESITY—Although precise definitions vary among experts, overweight has been traditionally defined as 10 to 20% above an optimal weight for height derived from statistics. Obesity is defined as body weight being 20% above normal. Some scientists argue that the amount and distribution of an individual's body fat is a significant indicator of health risk and therefore should be considered in defining overweight. Abdominal fat has been linked to more adverse health consequences than fat in the hips or thighs. Thus, calculations of waist-to-hip ratio are preferred by some health experts to help determine if an individual is overweight.

OMEGA-3 FATTY ACIDS—A type of fatty acid, commonly found in fish and fish oils. Omega-3 fatty acids consumed in moderate quantities are thought to reduce the risk of coronary artery disease in some individuals.

PHYTOCHEMICALS—A natural bioactive compound found in plant foods that works with nutrients and dietary fiber to protect against disease. Research suggests that phytochemicals, working together with nutrients found in fruits, vegetables, and nuts, may help slow the aging process and reduce the risk of many diseases, including cancer, heart disease, stroke, high blood pressure, cataracts, osteoporosis, and urinary tract infections.

POLYUNSATURATED FAT—A highly unsaturated fat found in food products derived from plants, including safflower, sunflower, corn, and soybean oils. Like monounsaturated fat, it is a healthier alternative to saturated fat.

POTASSIUM—Potassium is critical for maintaining a normal heart rhythm and mineral balance. Bananas are a good source of potassium. Cooked greens like spinach, baked sweet potato, and winter squash are vegetables that are also good sources.

PROTEIN—A large, complex molecule composed of amino acids. Proteins are essential to the structure, function, and regulation of the body. Examples are hormones, enzymes, and antibodies.

PROTEIN SOURCES—Nearly all animal foods, such as meat, dairy products, eggs, and fish are all concentrated sources of protein as they typically contain all nine essential amino acids. An often overlooked source of protein is plant foods; nuts, seeds, beans, and peas can be terrific sources of protein.

REGISTERED DIETICIAN—An authority on food and nutrition. The initials "RD" stand for Registered Dietitian. They have a minimum of a bachelor's degree, and many RDs have a master's degree or other advanced credentials, such as Certified Diabetes Educator (CDE) or Certified Nutrition Support Dietitian (CNSD). Dietitians may specialize in certain areas of nutrition including pediatric nutrition, diabetes, weight management, sports nutrition, digestive disorders, food allergies, geriatric nutrition, or eating disorders. RDs have successfully passed an extensive registration examination administered by the Commission on Dietetic Registration. All registered dietitians are required to complete at least 75 hours of continuing education every five years. In some states, dietitians are required to have a license.

RIBOFLAIN—Riboflavin helps the body break down carbohydrates, proteins and fats so they can be used for energy. It also is necessary for healthy skin, eyes, and clear vision.

SATURATED FATS—Saturated fats are found predominantly in animal products, including meat and dairy products. Some meats contain more saturated fat than others: beef more than chicken, for example. They are strongly associated with higher cholesterol level and have been associated with a higher risk for Type 2 diabetes. They may be even more dangerous in women than in men. The so-called tropical oils, palm, coconut, and cocoa butter, are also high in saturated fats.

SODIUM (SALT)—Sodium is a trace mineral that helps maintain body fluid balance. Most experts recommend salt restriction in people who are salt-sensitive. High-salt diets in anyone who is salt-sensitive may harm the heart, kidney, and brain and increase the risk for death, regardless of blood pressure. (Even people with normal blood pressure can be salt-sensitive.) Among those at highest risk for salt sensitivity are African Americans, people with diabetes, and the elderly.

SOLUBLE FIBER—A type of dietary fiber found in psyllium, cereals, oatmeal, apples, citrus fruits, beans, and other foods that increases the viscosity in the gut and acts to reduce high blood cholesterol levels, which decreases the risk of cardiovascular disease.

SOY PROTEIN—The protein found in soybeans and soy-based foods. It is rich in both soluble and insoluble fiber and omega-3 fatty acids, and provides all essential proteins. Studies have shown soy to reduce the cholesterol levels in people. Soy may also reduce other heart risk factors, including blood pressure, at least in certain populations.

STARCH SUGAR—Starch is a polymer or long string of glucose molecules, just as a protein is a long string of amino acids.

SUCROSE—A type of sugar. Sucrose is a diglyceride composed of glucose and fructose. Also, see "carbohydrates."

SUGAR—A class of carbohydrate with a characteristically sweet taste such as sucrose, raw sugar, turbinado sugar, brown sugar, honey, and corn syrup. A high level of sugar consumption has been associated with higher triglycerides and lower levels of HDL cholesterol, the so-called good cholesterol. The high consumption of sugar is most likely one of the factors in the current obesity epidemic. Soda, other sweetened beverages, and fruit juice may, in fact, be singled out as major contributors to childhood obesity.

SULFITES—Sometimes used to preserve the color of foods such as dried fruits and vegetables, and to inhibit the growth of microorganisms in fermented foods such as wine. Sulfites are safe for most people, however a small segment of the population has been found to develop shortness of breath or fatal shock shortly after exposure to these preservatives.

TOTAL FAT— Food labels and dietitians sometimes refer to a diet's total fat. Total fat refers to the amount of fat in the diet given as a percentage of total calories. It is recommended that 20% to 35% of your total calories come from fats. This includes all types of fats, including saturated, mono-unsaturated, and polyunsaturated fats.

TRANS-FATTY ACIDS—Manufactured fats created during a process called hydrogenation, which is aimed at stabilizing polyunsaturated oils to prevent them from becoming rancid and to keep them solid at room temperature. The main sources of trans-fatty acids in the American diet today are margarine, shortening, commercial frying fats and high-fat baked goods such doughnuts, crackers, white breads, and cookies. Trans-fatty acids, like saturated fats, raise blood LDL cholesterol levels (the so-called "bad" cholesterol). High consumption of trans-fatty acids may also reduce the HDL or "good" cholesterol levels. Some experts believe that these partially hydrogenated fats are even worse for the heart than saturated fats. They may also pose a risk for certain cancers.

TYPE 2 DIABETES—Non-insulin dependent (Type 2) diabetes is the more common type of diabetes. People of African-American, Hispanic, and Native American decent are at higher risk of this disease. The disease develops slowly and usually becomes evident after age 40. Being overweight is a common risk factor. Often it can be controlled through diet, weight control, and exercise.

UNSATURATED FATS—Unsaturated fats (e.g., monounsaturated and polyunsaturated fats), found mostly in plants, are liquid at room temperature. They are less likely to cause heart disease than saturated fats. Polyunsaturated fats are found in safflower, sunflower, corn, soybean, and cottonseed oils, and in some fish. Recent research shows that monounsaturated fats found in olive, peanut, and canola oils may even lower cholesterol.

VITAMIN A—Vitamin A is associated with eye health because it protects the surface of the cornea. It is essential for the development of bones, growth, and reproduction. It helps the body resist infection by protecting the linings of the respiratory, digestive, and urinary tracts and maintains healthy skin and hair. Good sources of vitamin A are liver and fish-liver oils, egg yolk, and milk and dairy products. Also know as beta-carotene, it is found in dark green leafy vegetables (like spinach and turnip greens), deep-yellow fleshed root vegetables (e.g. carrots, sweet potatoes), squash (acorn, butternut, etc.), some fruits (apricots), and red bell peppers.

VITAMIN B1—Also know as thiamine, vitamin B1 is involved in the functioning of the nerves, muscles, and heart, and the moderation of carbohydrates. The best sources of thiamine are whole grains and cereals, and enriched grain products (white flour and white rice are often enriched with the vitamin B complex and iron to replace some of the nutrients lost by processing). Other good sources are legumes (dried beans, peas, and nuts), organ meats, lean pork, and eggs.

VITAMIN B2—Also known as riboflavin, vitamin B2 is involved in the metabolism of carbohydrates, fats, and proteins; the utilization of other vitamins; the production of hormones from the adrenal gland; and eye and skin care. The best sources of riboflavin are organ meats, enriched breads and cereals, legumes, cheese, and eggs. Meat, fish, and dark-green vegetables are fairly good sources.

VITAMIN B3—Also known as niacin, vitamin B3 is involved in the metabolism of carbohydrates and fats, the functioning of the digestive system, the manufacture of sex hormones, and the maintenance of healthy skin. Niacin is found in a wide variety of foods, particularly meat, organ meats, whole grains and cereals, and legumes. Other sources are eggs, milk, green leafy vegetables, and fish.

VITAMIN B5—Also known as pantothenic acid, vitamin B5 is involved in the production of hormones in the adrenal gland and maintaining the body's immune system. It is also an essential factor in the release of energy from food. The best sources of pantothenic acid are organ meats, yeast, raw vegetables, eggs, and dairy products.

VITAMIN B6—Also known as pryidoxine, vitamin B6 is involved in the body's metabolism of protein, the formation of hemoglobin, the functioning of the digestive and nervous systems, and the maintenance of healthy skin. The best sources of pyridoxine are whole-grain products, poultry, fish, and nuts. Other good sources are meat, most fruits and vegetables, eggs, and dairy products.

VITAMIN B12—Vitamin B12 works with folic acid to build the genetic material of cells and produce blood cells in the bone marrow. It is also involved in activities of some of the body's enzymes (substances that promote chemical reactions in the body) and helps maintain a healthy nervous system. The best sources of vitamin B12 are organ meats. Fish (especially sardines, herring, and oysters), lean meats, poultry, cheese, and eggs are also good sources. The only known plant sources are yeast, alfalfa, and two Japanese seaweeds—wakame and kombu.

VITAMIN C—Vitamin C helps wounds heal, improves the body's absorption of iron, and is involved in the growth and maintenance of bones, teeth, gums, ligaments, and blood vessels. Vitamin C is found almost exclusively in fruits and vegetables. Breast milk and organ meats also contain small amounts. Tomatoes, peppers, cabbage, potatoes, and dark, leafy greens such as spinach, romaine lettuce, and watercress are all good sources of vitamin C, as well as oranges, grapefruit, cantaloupe, strawberries, and broccoli.

VITAMIN D—Vitamin D works with calcium to build strong bones and teeth and maintain the nervous system. Called the "sunshine vitamin," it can be manufactured in the body from exposure to sunlight—sun exposure is the primary source of vitamin D for most people. Food sources include egg yolk, liver, tuna, fatty fish such as herring, mackerel, and salmon; and vitamin D-fortified milk or juice.

VITAMIN E—Vitamin E is an antioxidant that helps protect the lungs, nervous system, skeletal muscles, and the eye retinas from damage by free radicals (cell-damaging chemicals). It also protects against cell damage and is believed to slow down the aging of cells. Sources of vitamin E include nuts, vegetable oils, egg yolks, whole-wheat products, and green leafy vegetables.

VITAMIN H—Also know as biotin, vitamin H is involved in the enzyme action that enables protein and carbohydrate metabolism, the breakdown of fatty acids, and the synthesis of DNA in cells. Foods rich in biotin include oats, organ meats, yeast, and eggs (cooked); smaller amounts are found in whole-wheat products, diary products, fish, and tomatoes.

VITAMIN K —Vitamin K is known to be needed to coagulate blood and to maintain proper bone density. It has been shown to help prevent degenerative diseases like osteoporosis and heart disease. Good sources of vitamin K include dark-green leafy vegetables, eggs, cheese, pork, and liver.

VITAMIN M—Folic acid is essential to many of the body's enzyme activities, including the synthesis of protein and the genetic materials RNA and DNA. Rich sources of folic acid include vegetables, organ meats, whole-wheat products, legumes, and mushrooms.

VITAMINS—Organic compounds that are nutritionally essential in small amounts to control metabolic processes. Most cannot be synthesized by the body. Vitamins are obtained from food, except for vitamin D and vitamin K, which the body can synthesize.

WATER—Although deficiencies of energy or nutrients can be sustained for months or even years, a person can survive only a few days without water. Experts rank water second only to oxygen as essential for life. In addition to offering true refreshment for the thirsty, water plays a vital role in all bodily processes.

WHOLE GRAINS—The whole kernel of grain that includes the bran (outer shell), germ (nutrient-rich core), and endosperm (starchy portion). The health benefit provided by whole grains is the reduced risk of cardiovascular disease, which results from the combination of fiber, vitamins, minerals, and phytochemicals found in whole grains.

Index

Fat Flush Diet 52
French Diet 62
Get With the Program Diet 65
Jorge Cruise Diet 90
Life Choice Diet 95
NutriSystem Diet 119
Peanut Butter Diet 125
Pritikin Diet 131
Revival Soy Diet 143
Richard Simmons Diet 145
Rosedale Diet 148
Scan Diet 152
Shape Up Diet 159
Somersizing Diet 166
Step Diet 177
Weight Watchers Diet 206

F

fasting 42, 46, 57, 201, 202, 203, 204,
    238, 248
Fats
    monounsaturated fats 73–75, 91,
        112, 113, 122, 125, 149, 169,
        173, 216, 217, 259, 260
    polyunsaturated fats 113, 122, 169,
        183, 224
    omega-3 fatty acids 73, 112, 113,
        114, 122, 123, 129, 131, 148,
        169, 217, 225, 228, 246, 250,
        257, 264, 265, 271
    omega-6 fatty acids 74, 122, 123,
        226, 250
    saturated fats 4, 14, 73–75, 91, 95,
        108, 112, 113, 122, 125, 128,
        129, 149, 169, 183, 216, 217,
        224, 231, 233, 245, 246, 256, 259
fatty fish 112, 123, 266
fish oils 73, 217
folic acid. *See* Vitamins
Food-Combining Diets
    Beverly Hills Diet 15
    Fit for Life Diet 56
    Hay Diet 76
    Somersizing Diet 166

food additives 42, 248, 254
food allergies 108
French paradox 62

G

gastroesophageal reflux disease 80,
    221
GERD 221
gluten 234
glycemic index 67, 68, 69, 83, 85, 128,
    170, 171, 172, 173, 182, 189, 259

H

Harvard School of Public Health 266
Healthy Food Pyramid 266
heartburn 221
high blood pressure 13, 14, 48, 102,
    136, 137, 157, 193, 194, 195,
    239, 260, 269, 271
High Protein Diets. *See* Low-Carbohy-
    drate Diets
hypertension (high blood pressure)
    63, 115, 123, 135, 264, 269, 271,
    272

I

IBS (irritable bowl syndrome) 79, 241
iron. *See* Minerals in food
isoflavones 143

K

ketones 10
ketosis 10, 11, 14, 40, 83, 84, 138, 155,
    173, 215
kidney disease 13, 14, 21, 40, 84, 85,
    137, 157, 173, 239, 247, 258

L

lactose intolerance 241, 243
lectins 18
Lipoproteins
    high-density lipoproteins 230
    low-density lipoproteins 230
Livatone powder 98